BRITISH COLUMBIA CANCER AGENCY
LIBRARY
600 WEST 10th AVE.
VANCOUVER, B.C. CANADA
V5Z 4E6

HANDBOOK OF
NUCLEAR MEDICINE

D0950456

HANDBOOKS IN RADIOLOGY SERIES

Other Volumes in This Series

HANDBOOK OF NUCLEAR MEDICINE

FREDERICK L. DATZ, M.D.
Professor of Radiology
Director of Nuclear Medicine
University of Utah School of Medicine
Salt Lake City, Utah

SECOND EDITION

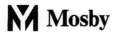 Mosby

St. Louis Baltimore Boston Chicago London Madrid Philadelphia Sydney Toronto

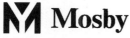

Dedicated to Publishing Excellence

Editors: Anne S. Patterson and Robert J. Farrell
Developmental Editor: Maura K. Lieb
Project Manager: Patricia Tannian
Production Editor: Mary McAuley
Senior Book Designer: Gail Morey Hudson
Manufacturing Supervisor: Theresa Fuchs

SECOND EDITION

Copyright © 1993 by Mosby–Year Book, Inc.

Previous edition copyrighted 1988

All rights reserved. No part of this publication may be reproduced, stored in a retrieval system, or transmitted, in any form or by any means, electronic, mechanical, photocopying, recording, or otherwise, without prior written permission from the publisher.

Permission to photocopy or reproduce solely for internal or personal use is permitted for libraries or other users registered with the Copyright Clearance Center, provided that the base fee of $4.00 per chapter plus $.10 per page is paid directly to the Copyright Clearance Center, 27 Congress Street, Salem, MA 01970. This consent does not extend to other kinds of copying, such as copying for general distribution, for advertising or promotional purposes, for creating new collected works, or for resale.

Printed in the United States of America
Composition by University Graphics, Inc.
Printing/binding by Malloy Lithographing, Inc.

Mosby-Year Book, Inc.
11830 Westline Industrial Drive, St. Louis, Missouri 63146

Library of Congress Cataloging in Publication Data
Datz, Frederick L.
    Handbook of nuclear medicine / Frederick L. Datz.—2nd ed.
    p.   cm.   — (Handbooks in radiology series)
    Rev. ed. of: Nuclear medicine. ©1988.
    Includes bibliographical references and index.
    ISBN 0-8016-7700-9
    1. Radioisotope scanning—Handbooks, manuals, etc. 2. Nuclear
medicine—Handbooks, manuals, etc. I. Datz, Frederick L. Nuclear
medicine. II. Title. III. Series.
    [DNLM: 1. Nuclear Medicine—handbooks. WN 39 D234n 1993]
RC78.7.R4D38   1993
616.07'575—dc20
DNLM/DLC
for Library of Congress   93-14365
                                                                CIP

93 94 95 96 97 / 9 8 7 6 5 4 3 2 1

To
Terry and Katie

Preface

The second edition of *Handbook of Nuclear Medicine* has the same purpose as the first: to serve as a review of nuclear medicine for residents and fellows and to be a practical reference for practicing physicians. To better meet these goals, I have added sections to the second edition on a variety of new subjects and have changed the emphasis in others to reflect current trends in nuclear medicine. The neuroimaging section emphasizes single photon emission computed tomography (SPECT) with new agents such as HMPAO; the discussion of conventional imaging is reduced to brain death and inflammatory diseases. An overview of positron emission tomography (PET) has been expanded. I have added discussions of sestamibi and teboroxime to the chapter on cardiac imaging, as well as a review of pharmacologic stress associated with dipyridamole and adenosine. The use of PET for cardiac imaging is also discussed. I have also added a review of computer-assisted cardiac diagnosis, which will play an increasingly important role in the future.

Other changes include updating the section on renal scanning to include MAG_3, captopril challenge for renovascular hypertension, and new techniques for the furosemide washout test and glomerular filtration rate determination. Antibody imaging for cancer and infection and new leukocyte imaging techniques with ^{99m}Tc HMPAO have been added to the chapter on hematologic imaging. The PIOPED results and interpretation scheme have been added to the chapter on pulmonary imaging. Most other sections, too, have been updated, and I have added new references to each chapter.

I have maintained the outline format to make the book easier to use. However, the format has been simplified to clarify the transition from one section to the next.

I appreciate the many thoughtful comments and helpful suggestions from readers. I hope you find the second edition useful in your studies and in the daily practice of nuclear medicine.

Frederick L. Datz, MD

Contents

1

Endocrine System Imaging

THYROID
Anatomy

I. Embryology.
- A. Thyroid has dual origin.
  1. Main anlage develops as median endodermal down growth from tongue (foramen cecum). Cell remnants along tract of lingual evagination often connect with thyroid to produce pyramidal lobe. Follicular cells of thyroid, cells responsible for production of thyroid hormones, are primarily derived from these cells.
  2. Lateral anlage developed from fourth pharyngeal pouches—ectoderm. Primarily responsible for development of parafollicular C cells, although probably contributes to formation of follicular cells as well.

II. Thyroid has shieldlike shape. Left and right lobes connected by isthmus and lie in front of trachea below thyroid cartilage.

III. Weight of gland is 15 to 25 g in normal adult.

IV. Variations in size and contour common.
- A. Right lobe usually larger than left. Extends more superiorly and inferiorly than left lobe. Ratio of projected area on anterior view: left/right—approximately 0.8.
- B. Pyramidal lobe present in approximately 35% of patients; most frequently arises from isthmus or adjacent portions of the lobes, more commonly left.
- C. Congenital absence of a lobe is a rare variation.
- D. Remnant attachment of foramen cecum of tongue to thyroid is thyroglossal duct. Remnants of functioning tissue along this tract may result in lingual or sublingual thyroid as well as pyramidal lobe. When lingual thyroid is present, it is usually the only functioning thyroid tissue present.
- E. Ectopic functioning thyroid tissue rarely is found in ovary—struma ovarii. Arises in teratogenic cysts. May produce thyrotoxicosis or become malignant.

Physiology

I. Thyrotropin-releasing hormone (TRH).
  A. Small tripeptide formed in hypothalamus. Flows along neurons to median eminence where it enters the hypophyseal portal system, which supplies the anterior pituitary. Here thyroid-stimulating hormone (TSH) is released after TRH stimulation. TSH directly stimulates release of hormones from thyroid. Note that strong feedback mechanism occurs with TRH. As triidothyronine (T_3) or thyroxine (T_4) level increases, TRH falls, decreasing TSH secretion.
II. Thyroid hormone produced as follows:
  A. Ingestion.
    1. Iodine ingested daily: 250 to 600 μg.
    2. Ingested iodine rapidly reduced to iodide in upper intestine.
    3. Absorption is 90% in the first 60 minutes after ingestion.
    4. Iodide distributed in blood as an extracellular ion similar to chloride.
    5. Leaves blood primarily via thyroid uptake; remainder by renal excretion.
  B. Iodide trapping.
    1. Thyroid pump, dependent on oxidative phosphorylation, permits intracellular concentrations of iodine of 30:1 in normal persons. May rise as high as 500:1 in disease states.
    2. Oxidative phosphorylation inhibitors reduce uptake:
      a. Cyanides.
      b. Dinitrophenol.
      c. Anoxia.
      d. Hypothermia.
    3. Iodine trapping can be competitively blocked by monovalent anions including:
      a. TcO_4^-—pertechnetate.
      b. CLO_4^-—perchlorate.
      c. SCN^-—thiocyanate.
    4. These agents return unbound thyroidal iodine to plasma, effectively "washing out" thyroidal iodine. Serves as basis of perchlorate washout test. Reflects iodine that has been trapped but has not been organified.
  C. Organification.
    1. Iodide is oxidized to iodine via peroxidase, which catalyzes the reaction of iodine with hydrogen peroxide.
    2. Following oxidation, iodine is incorporated into tyrosine to form monoiodotyrosine (MIT) and diiodotyrosine (DIT), which are bound to thyroglobulin.

3. Peroxidase abnormalities.
    a. Peroxidase deficiency causes congenital hypothyroidism.
    b. Pendred's syndrome—autosomal-recessive associated with normal peroxidase activity but deficient peroxide resulting in ineffective organification. These patients have combination of moderate hypothyroidism, goiter, and nerve deafness.
4. Propylthiouracil (PTU) and methimazole (Tapazole) prevent organification.

D. Coupling.
1. Coupling of MIT and DIT occurs by:
    a. Molecular rearrangement.
    b. Intermolecular transfer to form T_3 and T_4.
    c. Coupling appears to occur while tyrosine bound to thyroglobulin; catalyzed by thyroid peroxidase.

E. Storage.
1. Triiodothyronine and T_4 stored in thyroglobulin within follicles.

F. Release.
1. TSH binds to thyroid cell membrane, activating adenyl cyclase. Increase in cyclic adenosine monophosphate (c-AMP) results in hydrolysis of thyroglobulin releasing T_3 and T_4.
2. MIT and DIT released along with T_3 and T_4 when thyroglobulin undergoes proteolytic degradation.
3. MIT and DIT then deiodinated within thyroid gland by deiodinase (dehalogenase) and released iodine reutilized to synthesize more thyroid hormone precursors.
4. Deiodinase deficiency can cause hypothyroidism. Diagnosed by identifying labeled MIT and DIT in blood and urine of patients following administration of radioactive iodine.

G. Peripheral metabolism.
1. Triiodothyronine and T_4 bound in blood to:
    a. Thyroid-binding globulin (TBG) (70%).
        (1) T_4 strongly bound.
        (2) T_3 less strongly bound.
    b. Albumin (20%).
    c. Thyroid-binding prealbumin (TBPA) (10%).
        (1) T_3 weakly bound.
        (2) T_4 weakly bound.
2. Thyroxine converted peripherally to T_3, which is the tissue active hormone. T_4 is a prohormone. T_3 primarily derived from peripheral deiodination of T_4.

   3. Clearance half-times blood are:
      a. T_4—6 days.
      b. T_3—1 day.
   4. Peripherally circulating hormone responsible for increasing basal metabolic rate as well as having profound effect on growth and development.
   5. When TBG is low, bound serum T_4 concentration falls. (Normally <1% circulating T_4 is free—this small fraction is available to tissues to maintain metabolic balance.) Free T_4 usually maintained despite low TBG, so patients remain clinically euthyroid.
   6. PTU blocks peripheral conversion T_4 to T_3.
   7. End-organ resistance to thyroid hormone has been described in some children with goiter. They have a high concentration of T_4 with clinical euthyroidism.

Radiopharmaceuticals

  I. Technetium 99m pertechnetate.
     A. Decay—isomeric transition.
     B. Physical half-life—6 hours.
     C. Gamma energy—140-keV photon.
     D. 0.5% to 3.75% of administered dose taken up by 20 to 30 minutes. Therefore, higher doses must be used with pertechnetate than with iodine for adequate photon flux.
     E. Technetium is trapped but *not* organified. This can lead to discrepancy in scan results in chronic thyroiditis in which increased trapping occurs without organification, i.e., better technetium uptake than iodine uptake. This is diagnostic of thyroiditis in absence of drugs that block hormone synthesis such as PTU.
     F. There have been occasional reported cases of disparate images between iodine and pertechnetate in well-differentiated thyroid carcinomas, i.e., pertechnetate uptake equal to remainder of gland in face of cold nodule on iodine imaging. This again is caused by $^{99m}TcO_4^-$ trapping without organification. The frequency of disparate imaging in thyroid malignancy is thought to be infrequent, although estimates vary. Note that a cold nodule on technetium will be cold on iodine (although reverse disparity has also been reported).
     G. Dose—1 to 10 mCi (3 to 4 mCi usually adequate).
     H. Radiation dose—0.2 to 2 rad.
 II. Iodine 123.
     A. Decay—electron capture.
     B. Half-life—13 hours.

C. Gamma decay—159 keV.

D. Cyclotron produced.

E. Radiation exposure significantly increased if contaminated by other cyclotron-produced isotopes of iodine—especially ^{124}I. These isotopes have high-energy photons and longer half-lives, resulting in degradation of the thyroid images as well. Newer production techniques improve purity.

F. Dose—100 to 300 µCi.

III. Iodine 131.

A. Decay—beta, gamma.

B. Half-life—8.04 days.

C. Gamma photon—364 keV (82%); also 637-keV photon (6.8% of disintegrations).

D. Production—fission of ^{235}U or reactor—

$$^{130}\text{Te} \rightarrow {}^{131}\text{Te} \overset{\text{beta}}{\rightarrow} {}^{131}\text{I}.$$

E. ^{131}I has several disadvantages and is currently used only for uptakes, scanning for thyroid cancer, and therapy.

1. Radiation exposure extremely high—1 to 2 rad/µCi. This is related to beta emission (192-keV average).

2. High energy of principal gamma photon (364 keV) inefficiently collimated and detected by gamma cameras. (637-keV photon results in more severe septal penetration and image degradation.)

3. Long half-life makes suppression and serial studies difficult.

F. Dose.

1. Uptake—3–5 µCi.

2. Scanning—50–100 µCi. (Dose for thyroid imaging; cancer imaging doses are higher.)

IV. Iodine 125.

A. Decay—electron capture.

B. Half-life—60 days.

C. Gamma photon—27–35 keV.

D. Radiation dose—similar to ^{131}I.

E. Energy of photon and significant attenuation makes imaging with gamma cameras impossible. Primarily used in radioimmunoassay.

V. Thallium 201.

A. See Chapter 7.

B. Sometimes used for whole-body imaging in patients with thyroid carcinoma. Advantage is that patient does not need to be off suppression. Sensitivity for metastases is controversial. Some studies have shown better sensitivity than ^{131}I, others poor sensitivity. We have not had good success with ^{201}Tl.

Technique

I. Thyroid uptake.
  A. Thyroid uptake is percentage of administered radiopharmaceutical that is taken up by the thyroid over a specified period of time.
  B. An uptake probe (usually 5 × 5 cm NaI [Tl] crystal) with collimator is used with a thyroid-to-crystal distance of 35 cm.
  C. The patient's dose capsules, and a standard for quality control, are placed in a plastic neck phantom that corrects for attenuation by simulating thickness of the neck structures. These are counted at the same distance from the probe at which the patient will be counted.
  D. The capsules are orally administered to the patient.
  E. Uptakes are performed at 2 or 4 hours and again at 24 hours.
  F. Counts per minute (CPM) in the thyroid are obtained. Then, to correct for background in the blood in the neck, a second count is performed over the thigh, approximately 10 cm above the patella. In addition, the standard is recounted to check for equipment problems.
  G. The uptake is calculated as follows:

$$\% \text{ uptake} = \frac{\text{CPM thyroid} - \text{CPM thigh}}{\text{CPM dose administered} \times \text{decay factor}} \times 100$$

  Note that decay factor varies with the time of imaging and half-life of isotope used.
  H. Often, scattered photons with ^{123}I are more abundant than with ^{131}I. In addition, Compton plateau closer to ^{123}I photopeak. Therefore, any change in high voltage will have greater effect on ^{123}I recorded counts. In addition, downscatter from contaminants, such as ^{124}I, contribute to spectrum.
  I. Uptakes can be performed with ^{99m}Tc pertechnetate but are less accurate. This is due to:
    1. Low absolute uptake of pertechnetate.
    2. High neck background.
    3. Activity in neck constantly changing because of changes in biodistribution of pertechnetate. Pertechnetate usually bound to plasma proteins. Compartmental analysis shows 50% to 60% disappears in first few minutes; 15% T½, 5 to 7.5 minutes; 25% T½, 100 to 300 minutes.
    4. Material concentrated in salivary glands, gastric mucosa, choroid plexus. Excreted primarily in gastrointestinal (GI) tract (critical organ) and kidneys. In kidneys, excretion by filtration with 85% reabsorbed in tubules; 30% excreted in urine first 24-hour period, 40% excreted in fecal material over first 4 hours.

       5. Because of these problems, some advocate neck-to-thyroid ratios instead. Normal approximately 2.5 to 5.5.

II. Perchlorate washout test.
   - A. Used to diagnose organification defects such as in Hashimoto's thyroiditis or congenital enzyme deficiencies (peroxidase deficiency).
   - B. 20 μCi of ^{131}I administered orally.
   - C. Uptake measured 2 hours.
   - D. Patient given 1 g of potassium perchlorate orally. Perchlorate is trapped by thyroid and competitively displaces iodide that has not been organified.
   - E. Uptakes are performed every 15 minutes for 90 minutes after potassium perchlorate administration.
   - F. Normally no variation in thyroid activity found after perchlorate. Positive study if calculated uptake falls 15% below 2-hour value.

III. T_3 suppression test.
   - A. Used to diagnose borderline hyperthyroidism. This is done by showing the autonomy of the thyroid gland.
   - B. A radioiodine uptake is performed.
   - C. Patient is given 25 μg of T_3 orally three times a day for 7 days.
   - D. Uptake remeasured.
   - E. Normally, uptake falls greater than 60% below baseline value. Suppression does not occur in borderline hyperthyroidism.
   - F. Note that TRH stimulation test has largely replaced this test.

IV. Thyroid scan with ^{99m}Tc pertechnetate.
   - A. Inject 3–4 mCi of technetium pertechnetate intravenously (IV).
   - B. Wait 20 minutes before scanning.
   - C. Using a gamma camera equipped with a pinhole collimator, obtain 100,000 count anterior image. Obtain 30-degree left anterior oblique (LAO) and right anterior oblique (RAO) projections for the same time as anterior image.
   - D. Any nodules should be marked and additional views obtained.

 V. Thyroid scan with ^{123}I.
   - A. Administer 200 to 300 μCi of ^{123}I orally.
   - B. Image at 4 or 24 hours.
   - C. Using a gamma camera equipped with pinhole collimator, obtain 100,000 count images in the anterior projection. Obtain 30-degree LAO and 30-degree RAO views for the same length of time as the anterior image.
   - D. May obtain "pullback image" after other views to show mediastinum if substernal thyroid is a question.
   - E. Any nodules should be marked and additional views obtained.

VI. Fluorescent scanning.
   - A. Alternative type of thyroid scanning. Americium-241 source is

used to irradiate the thyroid with 59.6 KeV-gamma photon. This excites K-shell electrons of iodine via photoelectric interaction. A 28.5-KeV characteristic K x-ray is emitted. These x-rays are detected by a collimated solid-state lithium-doped silicon detector.

B. The scan reveals the distribution of stable iodine within the gland. Radiation exposure is extremely low:
   1. Thyroid—15 mrad.
   2. Whole body—0 mrad.
C. An advantage is that thyroid image can be obtained in patients whose iodine pool has been flooded with exogenous iodine.

Normal Scan

  I. Homogeneous uptake of the radiopharmaceutical.
 II. Common variations, as noted earlier, included a left lobe smaller than the right and a pyramidal lobe.
III. Lateral margins of the thyroid are usually straight or convex; concave borders should alert one to possibility of an internal or extrinsic mass.
 IV. On oblique images, position of the tracheal cartilage may create appearance of defect, especially in medial portion of contralateral lobe in region of isthmus.
  V. With pertechnetate, activity in esophagus may be seen. To differentiate from ectopic thyroid tissue, have patient drink glass of water and repeat imaging. Less commonly seen with iodine.
 VI. Studies of thyroid scans in asymptomatic patients undergoing pertechnetate scans for purposes other than thyroid imaging indicate high incidence of abnormalities. Specifically:
   A. 30%—inhomogeneity.
   B. 40%—irregularities of borders.
   C. Nodules.
      1. Single nodules—2.7%.
      2. Multiple nodules—26%.
      3. Note that incidence of nodules increases from 0% in first decade to 40% in those 51 to 80 years of age.

Abnormal Studies

  I. Nonvisualization of thyroid gland (low uptake).
   A. Increased iodine pool.
      1. Recent contrast media.
      2. Exogenous iodine.
         a. Kelp (present in some vitamins and health foods).
         b. Medications (Betadine, antipertusives, etc.).
   B. Ingestion of goiterogenic foods that liberate thiocyanates on

digestion. These materials compete with iodine for trapping. Examples:

1. Turnips.
2. Cabbage.

C. Antithyroid medication—propylthiouracil, methimazole.
D. Thyroiditis.
E. Hypothyroidism—primary, secondary, or tertiary.
F. Ectopic thyroid tissue.

II. Nodules.

A. General.
   1. Most frequent indications for thyroid scanning.
      a. One-quarter—solitary nodule.
      b. Three-quarter—multiple nodules.
   2. Common—50% of autopsied glands contain nodules.
   3. Note large number of thyroid nodules found with pertechnetate scanning (see above).
      a. Incidence of nodularity increases with age.
         1. Fifteen to 24 years of age—17.7%.
         2. Over 65 years of age—30.4%.
      b. Nodules are more common in females than males.

B. Cold nodules.
   1. Causes of a solitary cold nodule on thyroid scan are as follows:
      a. Adenoma.
      b. Adenomatous hyperplasia/colloid cyst.
      c. Primary thyroid carcinoma.
      d. Hematoma.
      e. Thyroiditis.
      f. Fibrosis.
      g. Extrinsic mass impinging on thyroid.
   2. Scan sensitivity related to nodule size.
      a. 6.6 mm to 1 cm—56%.
      b. 1.2 cm—92%.
      c. >2 cm—100%.
   3. Risk of malignancy—10% to 20%.
   4. Malignant risk increased if:
      a. Occurs in male.
      b. Occurs in individual <40 years old.
      c. Enlarges even in the face of suppression.
      d. History of radiation exposure.
      e. Symptomatic—i.e., vocal cord paralysis, Horner's syndrome, or dysphagia.
   5. Risk of malignancy decreased in:

a. Nodules that involve an entire lobe—more likely caused by thyroiditis.

b. Large soft nodules with smooth borders.

c. Nodules too small to be delineated by imaging.

d. Enlarged lobe without a change in image density.

e. Peripherally located nodules causing only slight replacement of normal tissue.

6. Multiple cold nodules.

   a. Causes.

      (1) Multinodular goiter.

      (2) Postirradiation—neoplasms.

      (3) Causes of solitary lesions listed above.

   b. Risk of carcinoma—controversial.

      (1) Significantly less than with solitary lesion.

      (2) Histologically—4% to 17%; however, clinically much lower.

7. Individuals with history of head and neck radiation.

   a. Patients who received head or neck irradiation for such benign conditions as thymic enlargement, hypertrophy of tonsils, or acne, for example, are at higher risk for development of thyroid carcinoma. Approximately 5% to 7% of patients so treated will develop thyroid cancer compared with 1/27,000 individuals in general population. Those irradiated at age <6 years at greatest risk.

   b. Average latency for development is 20 years (range—5 to 50+ years).

   c. Incidence of thyroid cancer increases with increasing doses of thyroidal radiation from 6.5 to 1500 rad. Although there is no threshold level of radiation, curve does not deviate from level with doses less than 6.5 rad. At higher doses, gland is destroyed and hypothyroidism, rather than cancer, results.

   d. Approximately 20% of patients will develop some type of thyroid abnormality.

   e. Nodules.

      (1) Thyroid cancer—30%.

      (2) Benign causes—70%.

          (a) Adenomatous hyperplasia.

          (b) Follicular adenoma.

          (c) Colloid cysts.

          (d) Thyroiditis.

      (3) Note that in many patients more than one type of pathologic change is present.

(4) Multiple cold defects do *not* reduce chance of thyroid carcinoma as in nonirradiated population; 40% of patients with multiple nodules will have thyroid cancer.

(5) Malignancies involved are the same as in nonirradiated populations, primarily papillary and follicular carcinoma. These tumors are *not* any more aggressive than tumors in nonirradiated patients.

(6) Role of thyroid scanning:

(a) Thyroid scanning finds 96% of nodules, whereas palpation finds only 60%.

(b) Frequency of malignancy in nonpalpable lesions detected only by thyroid imaging—20%.

(c) One quarter of patients with palpable or scintigraphic abnormalities, which themselves prove to be benign, have microscopic foci of cancer elsewhere in the thyroid gland. Clinical significance of these small tumors is unknown.

f. Follow-up of patients with history of head and neck irradiation:

(1) Begins with careful palpation and pertechnetate or ^{123}I thyroid scan.

(2) If negative, should have yearly follow-up by palpation. Controversial whether thyroid scan should be performed at yearly intervals as well.

(3) If scan is definitely abnormal, even in absence of palpable findings, many believe patients should definitely undergo surgery, since likelihood of having carcinoma is same as in patient with palpable cold nodule in the nonirradiated group.

(4) In case of patients with diffuse enlargement by palpation without palpable nodules, if scan normal (negative for nodules), patient should be placed on suppression and be reexamined at 6 months. If scan shows definite cold area but no nodule palpable, patient should be placed on thyroid hormone and be reexamined at 6 months. Surgical exploration not indicated until or unless nodule becomes palpable. Likely, these patients have either benign hypertrophy or Hashimoto's thyroiditis.

(5) In experimental animals, suppression with T_4 (reducing TSH stimulation on the thyroid) reduces chances of development of thyroid cancer postirradiation; may be useful in humans.

III. Thyroiditis.
   A. Acute thyroiditis.
      1. Extremely rare.
      2. Bacterial infection—staphylococcus, streptococcus, etc.
      3. Signs and symptoms.
         a. Pain.
         b. Chills and fever.
         c. Hot, tender, enlarged gland.
         d. Usually no signs or symptoms of hyperthyroidism or hypothyroidism.
      4. Level of T_4—normal; ^{131}I uptake—usually normal, may be low.
   B. Subacute thyroiditis (de Quervain's thyroiditis).
      1. Etiology unknown. Tendency for subacute thyroiditis to follow upper respiratory tract infections (URIs) or sore throats has suggested viral infection or immune reaction. Mumps virus implicated in some cases.
      2. Signs and symptoms.
         a. Pain and tenderness in thyroid region.
         b. Mild to moderate fever.
         c. Symptoms of thyrotoxicosis.
      3. Pathologic findings—mixture of subacute, chronic, granulomatous inflammation. Polymorphonuclear leukocytes (PMNs), lymphocytes, macrophages all present. Most distinctive feature is granuloma with giant cells clustered about degenerating thyroid follicles.
      4. Laboratory findings.
         a. Elevated erythrocyte sedimentation rate (ESR).
         b. Elevated T_4.
         c. Decreased ^{131}I uptake in presence of elevated T_4.
         d. Decreased or nonvisualization of gland on scan.
      5. Timing—onset over 1 to 2 weeks with disease fluctuating for additional 3 to 6 weeks. Several recurrences of diminishing intensity may extend over many months.
      6. Up to 10% of patients may become hypothyroid over the long term.
   C. Chronic thyroiditis.
      1. Hashimoto's thyroiditis.
         a. Etiology—autoimmune. Coexistence of Hashimoto's is frequent in other autoimmune diseases such as:
           (1) Pernicious anemia.
           (2) Sjögren's syndrome.

      (3) Systemic lupus erythematosus.

      (4) Rheumatoid arthritis.

      (5) Addison's disease.

  b. Marked familial incidence.

  c. Pathologic findings—lymphocytic cellular infiltration with fibrosis. Foreign-body giant cells and granulomas *not* present.

  d. Incidence—equal to Graves' disease, 3 to 6 per 10,000 diagnosed. Probably exists with much more frequency than diagnosed clinically.

  e. Usually affects females aged 30 to 50 years.

  f. Signs and symptoms.

      (1) Painless enlargement of the neck.

      (2) Rarely patient presents with the symptoms of hyperthyroidism in acute phase.

      (3) Firm, rubbery, enlarged gland by palpation.

  g. Twenty percent of patients have mild hypothyroidism at time of presentation. This is the more chronic phase.

  h. Laboratory findings.

      (1) Level of T_4—low to high, although typically in normal or low range.

      (2) Elevated antithyroglobulin and antimicrosomal antibodies.

      (3) Uptake of ^{131}I variable—depends on stage of disease. Usually uptake normal or low if patient hypothyroid. Note that due to organification defect associated with Hashimoto's disease, 2-hour uptake may be elevated in face of lower 24-hour uptake. This can be reflected by better visualization on pertechnetate than iodine scan.

      (4) Scan findings variable.

        (a) Frequently patchy uptake.

        (b) Single cold defect.

        (c) Multiple cold defects.

        (d) Scattered hot/cold defects with hot areas representing hyperplasia.

        (e) Poor thyroid visualization.

        (f) Normal appearance.

2. Reidel's thyroiditis or struma.

  a. Etiology unknown.

  b. Incidence—rare; 50 times less frequent than Hashimoto's thyroiditis.

    c. Primarily affects women in 30- to 60-year age group.

    d. Physical examination—thyroid normal or enlarged—extremely hard.

    e. Pathologically is a chronic sclerosing thyroiditis, with the gland being replaced by dense fibrosis with scattered solitary follicular cells and occasional acini. Fibrosis extends to bind thyroid firmly to trachea and strap muscles.

    f. Symptoms.

       (1) Usually related to local pressure.

          (a) Dyspnea.

          (b) Dysphagia.

          (c) Hoarseness.

          (d) Stridor—if pressure on recurrent laryngeal nerves.

    g. Laboratory findings: level of T_4 and ^{131}I uptake usually normal; depressed as more thyroid gland is destroyed.

    h. Disease may remain stable or progress slowly to produce hypothyroidism.

IV. Graves' disease.

  A. Etiology.

    1. Autoimmune disease in which antibodies bind to TSH receptors of thyroid cells stimulating gland hypertrophy, and increasing synthesis and secretion of thyroid hormone.

    2. Incidence—common; five times more common in women than in men. Peaks in third and fourth decades, although may occur at any age.

  B. Signs and symptoms.

    1. Specific signs of Graves' disease are due to excessive deposition of mucopolysaccharides.

      a. Exophthalmos.

      b. Pretibial myxedema.

      c. Acropachy—clubbing of terminal phalanges.

    2. Nonspecific symptoms result from hyperthyroidism.

      a. Central nervous system (CNS).

        (1) Nervousness.

        (2) Emotional lability.

        (3) Tremor.

      b. Cardiovascular.

        (1) Palpitation/tachycardia.

        (2) Skin.

          (a) Hot, moist skin (increased sweating, vasodilation).

        (b) Thinning of hair and nails, hair loss.

        (c) Heat intolerance.

    c. Gastrointestinal.

       (1) Weight loss in presence of good appetite.

       (2) Diarrhea.

    d. Reproductive.

       (1) Menses—irregular.

C. Laboratory findings.

  1. Elevated thyroid function tests.

  2. Increased uptake—in a few patients uptake will be normal (euthyroid Graves' disease—though may have exophthalmos).

D. Scan.

  1. Increased uptake.

  2. Diffuse homogeneous uptake.

  3. Prominent pyramidal lobe.

  4. In a few patients, gland will not be enlarged.

  5. 2.7% of patients with Graves' disease have cool or cold nodules (Marine-Lenhart syndrome). More radioresistant than Graves' disease.

E. Treatment.

  1. Drug therapy.

    a. Permanent remission rate low—25+%. Best response in:

       (1) Younger patients.

       (2) Smaller glands.

       (3) Milder disease.

       (4) Disease of short duration.

    b. Adverse reactions.

       (1) Rash.

       (2) Pruritus.

       (3) Leukopenia.

  2. Surgery.

    a. Permanent remission—85%.

    b. Complications.

       (1) 15% of patients relapse.

       (2) Hypothyroidism—25% at 10 years.

       (3) Hypoparathyroidism.

       (4) Recurrent laryngeal nerve paralysis.

  3. Radioiodine therapy.

    a. Theory.

       (1) Radioiodine taken up and held within cell or follicular lumen for significant time (effective half-life, 3 to 5 days).

(2) 606-KeV maximum energy beta particles produce major dose to thyroid tissue.

(3) Energy causes ionization and chromosomal damage, causing cells to lose ability to replicate.

b. Safety.

(1) Fifty years' experience with treatment.

(2) National Center for Radiologic Health study of 36,000 patients treated for hypothyroidism with ^{131}I, surgery, or antithyroid drugs.

(a) No increased incidence of leukemia. (Note that Graves' disease, by itself, has a 50% increased risk for leukemia.)

(b) No increased risk of thyroid cancer; in fact, at lowest risk of thyroid cancer, since radiation damages cells inhibiting replication.

(i) ^{131}I therapy—0.1% incidence thyroid cancer.

(ii) Medical—0.3%.

(iii) Surgical—0.5%.

c. Genetics/reproduction.

(1) 10-mCi dose with 75% uptake gives 2- to 3-rad ovarian dose.

(2) Maximum increased risk of a harmful genetic defect resulting from this radiation exposure would be 0.003% or less (note spontaneous risk is 0.8%).

(3) Follow-up of patients treated for hyperthyroidism and treated with much larger doses for thyroid cancer shows no increased incidence of infertility or genetic abnormalities.

(4) Pregnancy.

(a) Contraindication for ^{131}I therapy.

(b) After 12 weeks, fetus has formed thyroid tissue and can take up ^{131}I, which crosses placenta. Produces cretinism/congenital hypothyroidism.

(c) Therapy in first 12 weeks also contraindicated, since radiation to whole body of fetus is not recommended. PTU and, rarely, surgery, are primary forms of therapy in pregnancy.

d. Dose calculation.

(1) Individual.

(a) Required dose =

$$\text{thyroid (g)} \times \frac{\mu\text{Ci}}{\text{g}} \times \frac{100}{\%\text{ uptake}}$$

(b) Range, in general, is 80 to 160 µCi/g. Note that

approximately 80 to 100 µCi/g delivers between 5000 and 10,000 rad.

  (c) Problems in this approach:

    (i) Inability to precisely determine gland weight.

    (ii) Variations in biologic half-life of radiopharmaceutical in thyroid.

    (iii) Variations in radiosensitivity.

      a Recent studies have indicated poor success rate in preventing hypothyroidism and yet still being effective with individualized doses.

(2) Fixed.

  (a) Low dose—3 to 5 mCi administered as a fixed dose. Since initial onset of hypothyroidism is dose-related, has lower incidence of hypothyroidism. However, cure rate is lowered, as well.

  (b) High dose—fixed, 8- to 10-mCi dose given to all patients. Success rate with one therapy using this dosage range: >90%. Increased incidence of early onset hypothyroidism, however.

(3) Effect.

  (a) Earliest onset of effect is 2 to 6 weeks after administration. Patient's goiter will shrink and symptoms will decrease; average time for euthyroidism is 2 to 6 months. The delayed effect is due to:

    (i) Cells retain some function, although can't replicate after iodine therapy.

    (ii) Stored hormone needs to be metabolized.

  (b) Usually 3 months is the earliest that retreatment would be performed. some prefer to wait 1 year.

  (c) Beta blockers do not affect radioiodine treatment.

(4) Complications.

  (a) Hypothyroidism—main complication.

    (i) Dose-related; however, even with low doses, 76% of patients have hypothyroidism by 11 years posttreatment.

    (ii) Range in first year varies between 5% and 70%. Average approximately 5.5% per month for first 6 months; 1.3% per month for second 6 months.

    (iii) After that, rate is 2% to 6% per year (average 2.8% per year).

(b) Increased release of thyroid hormone.
   (i) Exacerbation of symptoms may occur because of release of stored hormone from radiation thyroiditis. May occur any time from 12 hours to 20 days after therapy, average 10 to 14 days.
   (ii) Thyroid stores can be lowered before radiation treatment in older patients, especially those with cardiovascular symptoms, who are most prone to thyroid storm. Prior therapy with a propylthiouracil to decrease stored hormone is performed. May discontinue drug therapy for approximately 2 days to treat with radioiodine. Propylthiouracil and/or beta blockers started 3 to 5 days after therapy.

V. Multinodular goiter (Plummer's disease).
   A. Etiology—may be related to iodine deficiency. In addition, frequently familial.
   B. Lifelong condition beginning in adolescence.
   C. Frequently presents as increased size of thyroid. There may be symptoms related to size increase.
   D. Development of hyperthyroidism is related to duration of goiter. Average duration before onset is 17 years. Note that 60% of patients over 60 years of age are thyrotoxic with multinodular goiter.
   E. Frequency of association of thyroid cancers is somewhat unclear. In surgical specimens, between 4% and 17% have been found to harbor carcinoma. However, this does not fit the number of clinical cases seen. It appears that carcinoma is unlikely to be associated in multinodular goiter.
   F. Scan findings.
      1. Multiple hot and cold nodules.
      2. Suppression of the remainder of the gland.
      3. Nodules not suppressed by T_3 administration.
      4. Administration of TSH causes suppressed areas to appear.
      5. Uptake elevated or normal (approximately 50%), even in the face of hyperthyroidism.
   G. Therapy.
      1. See Graves' disease. Note that multinodular goiter has greater radioresistance than Graves'. It appears that there are areas of low functional activity at the time of therapy that may become activated following destruction of hyperfunc-

tioning tissue. Therefore, larger doses of ^{131}I are employed. Note that induction of hypothyroidism after ^{131}I therapy is rare in this disease.

VI. Solitary hyperfunctioning adenoma (toxic adenoma).

   A. Similar to multinodular goiter. Higher doses of ^{131}I necessary for treatment. Induction of hypothyroidism rare.

   B. Note that, in general, nodule must be 2½ to 3 cm in size to produce hyperthyroidism.

VII. Thyroid cancer.

   A. Types.

      1. Papillary carcinoma.

         a. Most common type of thyroid carcinoma.

         b. May be pure papillary or contain follicular elements.

         c. Often multifocal.

         d. Prognosis–worse in:

            (1) Older patients.

               (a) Females >50 years of age; males >40 years of age.

            (2) Males have three times more malignant tumor by histologic grade.

            (3) Larger primary lesion (>5 cm).

            (4) Initial regional invasion.

            (5) Local recurrence.

            (6) Distant metastases.

               (a) Note that local nodal metastasis is common, (50% to 90%), especially in younger patients, decreases with age, and does not appear to influence survival.

               (b) Metastases to lung, bone, and brain at time of presentation occur in less than 1% of patients.

               (c) Distant metastases develop in 4% to 25% of patients.

            (7) Excellent overall prognosis; Massaferri reported 1% mortality over 10 years.

            (8) Prognosis especially good for occult or minimal disease, i.e., tumors less than 1.5 cm in diameter without metastases. Note that when local lymph node metastases are present in these patients, the recurrence rate increases, although the mortality does not. These patients can probably be treated more conservatively, that is, by means of partial thyroidectomy without ^{131}I therapy.

      2. Follicular carcinoma.

a. Represents 10% to 20% of thyroid cancers.
b. Commonly unifocal.
c. Occurs in older age group than does papillary.
d. Usually larger in size (tumors <2 cm are rare).
e. Regional lymph node metastases uncommon (10%).
f. Hematogenous dissemination to bone and lung occurs more frequently than with papillary carcinoma.
g. Prognosis worse with follicular carcinoma than with papillary. Angioinvasive disease has 10-year survival of 34% as opposed to the 97% survival for noninvasive disease.
h. Remainder of prognostic factors are the same as for papillary.
i. Note: Cannot use less than 1.5-cm tumor size as an excellent prognostic sign, since these tumors can become angioinvasive even when small.
j. Three percent of patients have metastases at the time of presentation.
k. Higher incidence of distant metastases during course of disease than with papillary.
3. Hürthle cell tumor (follicular variant).
a. Occurs in older age groups.
b. Distant metastasis common and slowly progressive.
c. Rarely demonstrates ^{131}I uptake.
4. Medullary carcinoma.
a. Uncommon.
b. Arises from parafollicular or C cells, which are responsible for secretion for calcitonin.
c. Tumors may present as headache and intractable diarrhea, since secrete number of substances, including histamine, serotonin, prostaglandin, and adrenocorticotropin (ACTH).
d. Familial variety—multiple endocrine neoplasia, type II, Sipple's syndrome, consists of:
(1) Medullary thyroid carcinoma.
(2) Bilateral phenochromocytomas.
(3) Parathyroid adenomas—hyperplasia.
(4) Neurofibromas and café au lait spots.
(5) Mucosal neuromas.
(6) Greatly reduced calcitonin levels.
e. Since these tumors are not derived from follicular cells, as as are papillary and follicular carcinoma, they will not concentrate ^{131}I.
f. ^{201}Thallium, ^{99m}Tc sestamibi, ^{131}I metaiodobenzylguani-

dine (MIBG), and ^{99m}Tc DMSA have all been used to localize medullary metastases. Exact mechanism of uptake is unclear.

5. Anaplastic carcinoma.
   a. Two histologic types.
      (1) Small cell.
      (2) Giant cell—more undifferentiated and more malignant type.
      (3) Due to undifferentiated nature of tumor, rarely takes up ^{131}I.
      (4) Extremely poor prognosis, especially for giant-cell type.

B. Diagnosis.
   1. Cannot detect metastases while thyroid is in place. Any iodine given is taken up by normal thyroid.
   2. After thyroidectomy, patient is given T_3 for 4 weeks and then no medication for 2 weeks. TSH determination is obtained; when over 30 to 50 IU/ml, thyroid scan is performed.
   3. Patient is given 2 to 10 mCi of ^{131}I orally (note that number of metastases detected will increase with increasing dosage).
   4. Whole-body scan is performed 48 to 72 hours later.
   5. It is common to see uptake in the neck postoperatively. This may represent local tumor, residual thyroid, or local nodal metastasis.
   6. Uptake in following structures is normal.
      a. Salivary glands.
      b. Gastrointestinal tract.
      c. Liver—occurs because of breakdown of radioiodinated thyroid proteins from residual thyroid or well-differentiated cancer.
      d. Kidneys.
      e. Bladder.
   7. Thallium scan.
      a. Whole-body thallium scans more sensitive than ^{131}I in some studies. European study shows twice the sensitivity of ^{131}I.
      b. United States studies have shown sensitivity of only 50%. Note that when both ^{131}I and thallium scanning were performed, virtually all cases were detected.
      c. One advantage of thallium is that patient does not need to be off suppression.
      d. Not commonly used to replace ^{131}I in the United States.
   8. Thyroglobulin.

    a. Thyroglobulin level is very low or undetectable in patients who do not have functioning tissue or metastases.

    b. Elevation of thyroglobulin level indicates local recurrence or metastases.

    c. Sensitivity of thyroglobulin has varied. Some studies have reported higher sensitivity than ^{131}I scanning, others have been less successful. Most centers combine thyroglobulin measurement with ^{131}I scanning.

C. Therapy.

  1. Used to ablate residual thyroid and to treat local tumor and metastases.

  2. Majority favor ablation of residual thyroid for several reasons:

    a. Allows accurate diagnosis of recurrence or metastases with ^{131}I scanning.

    b. Allows accurate monitoring with thyroglobulin levels.

    c. May reduce local recurrences or later metastases in cases of multifocal thyroid cancer.

  3. Ablative dose necessary is controversial.

    a. Doses of 30 to 150 mCi are commonly given. Higher doses can cause radiation thyroiditis. Note that large amounts of normal thryoid tissue are difficult to ablate. Repeat surgery is necessary in those cases.

  4. Low-iodine diet may be of value before treatment. However, diet appears to increase whole-body retention of iodine, thereby increasing whole-body radiation dose rather than selectively increasing biologic half-time in tumor.

  5. Treating local recurrences and metastases.

    a. Since most patients die of local invasion, it is important to adequately treat these patients.

    b. Survival with distant metastases is significantly decreased.

      (1) Lung metastases—87% survival at 10 years with therapy.

      (2) Bone metastases—44% survival at 10 years with therapy.

    c. Usual therapy doses:

      (1) Local disease in neck—150 mCi.

      (2) Lung metastases—175 mCi.

      (3) Bone metastases—200 mCi.

    d. Note that some attempt to calculate dose is based on a maximum dose of 200 rad to the blood and blood-forming elements. Using this technique, doses can vary between 70 and 600 mCi (average, 300 mCi).

  6. Complications.

      a. Leukemia.
        (1) Rare.
        (2) Found in older individuals treated at very frequent intervals with extremely high cumulative doses (900 mCi).
      b. Breast cancer—rare.
      c. Bladder cancer—rare.
      d. Bone marrow depression.
        (1) Transient anemia develops in 36% 4 to 8 weeks after therapy.
        (2) 10%—leukopenia.
        (3) 3%—thrombocytopenia.
        (4) Note that permanent bone marrow suppresion is rare.
      c. Sialoadenitis.
        (1) Leads to dry mouth.
        (2) Can be partially prevented by having patient suck on hard candies to increase salivary flow during therapy.
      d. Nausea and vomiting.
        (1) Frequently occur within first 12 hours of therapy.
        (2) May be related to radiation effects.
        (3) From 35% to 75% of patients become symptomatic.
        (4) Can pretreat with antiemetics to reduce incidence.
      e. Lung fibrosis.
        (1) Concern that patient with diffuse pulmonary metastases might develop pulmonary fibrosis after therapy.
        (2) Controversial, but appears that, with single dose, cannot have enough uptake to cause pulmonary fibrosis.
      f. Fertility and birth defects—33 children treated at 14 years of age with mean dose of 196 mCi did not develop infertility or increased birth defects. However, because of small size of study group, it is likely that small increases could not be detected.

PARATHYROID
Anatomy

  I. Embryology.
    A. Superior parathyroids originate in fourth branchial cleft. During fetal development, superior glands descend along with thyroid.
    B. Inferior parathyroids originate in third branchial cleft and descend along with thymus. Because of the greater distance they migrate, inferior glands tend to be more variable in location (see below).

II. Location.
   A. Superior parathyroids—99% located either behind upper pole of thyroid lobes or adjacent to cricoid cartilage.
   B. Inferior glands—much more variable location. Locations include:
      1. 57%—in region of inferior pole of thyroid.
      2. 39%—superior pole of thymus.
      3. 2%—mediastinum.
      4. 2%—other ectopic sites. Parathyroids may be found anywhere from angle of mandible to level of aortic arch. Ectopic glands commonly located:
         a. Lateral to thyroid.
         b. Retropharyngeal.
         c. Retroesophageal.
         d. Mediastinum and thymus.
III. More than four glands identified in 2.5% of patients.
IV. Average weight, 35 to 50 mg.
 V. When parathyroid glands become enlarged, such as from tumor or hyperplasia, inferior glands tend to extend into posterior mediastinum or descend along inferior thyroid veins into anterior mediastinum.

Physiology

 I. Main function of parathyroid is to synthesize, store, and secrete parathyroid hormone (PTH).
II. PTH regulates level of calcium and phosphorous in blood by:
   A. Increasing osteoclast activity or increasing release of ionic calcium from bone.
   B. Decreasing excretion of calcium in the kidney (increasing excretion of phosphates, sodium, and potassium).
   C. Acting indirectly with vitamin D to increase intestinal absorption of calcium.

Radiopharmaceuticals

 I. Thallium 201 (^{201}Tl).
   A. Cause of uptake by parathyroid tissue unknown. There are two possibilities:
      1. Increased blood flow to adenomatous or hyperplastic tissue— most likely explanation.
      2. Increased uptake of thallium as potassium analogue—less likely explanation; appears to be inverse relationship between serum potassium and uptake.
   B. (See Chapter 7 for further information.)
II. Technetium 99m (^{99m}Tc).
   A. ^{201}Tl also taken up by normal thyroid tissue, therefore technetium

scan performed and subtracted from thallium to see if any additional tissue present.

   B. (See "Thyroid Imaging" section.)

Technique

  I. ^{201}Tl/^{99m}Tc Dual radiotracer.

    A. Patient placed on imaging table, neck extended as in thyroid scan.

    B. Large-field-of-view camera with parallel-hole collimator interfaced to computer system is placed over the patient.

    C. Patient is injected with 2 mCi of ^{201}Tl intravenously (IV). After 5- to 30-minute delay, mediastinal view is obtained for 100,000 counts.

    D. Collimator is switched to a pinhole, and images of the neck are obtained for 100,000 counts.

    E. ^{99m}Tc pertechnetate scan performed in same position.

    F. Computer subtraction of images performed after count normalization.

    G. Note that the thallium scan should be performed first, since downscatter of technetium into thallium window can obscure lesion.

  II. ^{99m}Tc sestamibi.

    A. Can be used as a substitute for ^{201}Tl with a protocol similar to above.

    B. Can also be used by itself.

      1. Patient is injected with 20-25 mCi of ^{99m}Tc sestamibi IV.

      2. A large-field-of-view camera with a low-energy, high resolution parallel-hole collimator is used.

      3. Anterior images with the head and neck extended are done for 10 minutes.

      4. Two sets of images are obtained, one at 10 to 15 minutes after injection and the other at 2 to 3 hours.

    C. (See Chapter 7 for discussion of sestamibi.)

Findings

I. Hyperparathyroidism.

    A. Background.

      1. Occurs in 1 of 700 people. 70% female. Average age, 56 years. Extremely rare in children.

      2. Causes.

        a. 90%—single benign adenoma.

        b. 5%—secondary hyperplasia (resulting from renal failure or malabsorption).

        c. 4%—primary hyperplasia.

       d. 1%—parathyroid carcinoma.
    3. Adenomas larger in size than hyperplasia. This affects sensitivity (see below).
  B. Scan findings.
    1. ^{201}Tl/^{99m}Tc dual radiotracer.
       a. Area of increased uptake of ^{201}Tl remaining outside thyroid (i.e., not associated with normal thyroid tissue).
    2. ^{99m}Tc sestamibi.
       a. Dual radiotracer—findings similar to those with ^{201}Tl and ^{99m}Tc.
       b. Sestamibi alone—washout of the diffuse thyroid activity with a focal area of increased activity present on the delayed images.
  C. Sensitivity—overall, 80% to 90%; sensitivity depends on:
    1. Location.
       a. Ectopic tissue found best.
    2. Size.
       a. Masses <500 mg infrequently found.
       b. 500 to 1,500 mg—70% to 80% sensitivity.
       c. Masses >1,500 mg—100% sensitivity.
    3. Type of tissue.
       a. Hyperplastic glands found much less frequently than adenomas. Appears to be size related because, hyperplastic glands smaller (however, those due to renal failure often larger).
  D. Efficacy.
    1. 90% to 95%. Patients cured with one operation.
    2. Reason for imaging is to reduce surgical time and find ectopic glands. Note that 70% of missed adenomas found at reexploration were ectopic.

^{131}I MIBG SCANNING FOR PHEOCHROMOCYTOMAS
Anatomy

I. Embryology.
  A. Occur in 0.01% to 0.001% of the adult population. In hypertensives the incidence is higher, approximately 0.1%.
  B. Most commonly presents in fourth to fifth decades; 10% occur in children.
  C. Pheochromocytoma is a neuroectodermal tumor arising from chromaffin cells of the sympathetic adrenal system.
  D. Cells of the neural crest migrate from the thoracic region to form the sympathetic chain and other ganglia and to invade the developing adrenal cortex, where they become the adrenal medulla.

E. In childhood, extra-adrenal chromaffin tissue is abundant. From the age of 3, extra-adrenal sites regress, and in the adult chromaffin tissue is found primarily in the adrenal gland itself. Persistent extra-adrenal sites include the sympathetic ganglia and carotid bodies. Extra-adrenal "rests" of chromaffin tissue may persist in later life and become sites of extra-adrenal pheochromocytoma anywhere from the base of the skull to the bladder.

II. Location.

    A. In adults, 90% occur within the adrenal medulla. Thus, 10% are extra-adrenal. In children, a higher percentage, as many as 30%, are extra-adrenal.

Physiology

I. Biochemistry.

    A. Catecholamines are produced by these tumors.

    B. Epinephrine-secreting tumors are usually found within the adrenal glands, whereas norepinephrine may be secreted by either intra-adrenal or extraadrenal tumors. This is related to the enzyme phenyl-ethanolamine-N-methyltransferase (PNMT), which is found predominantly in the adrenal medulla and converts norepinephrine to epinephrine.

Clinical Features

I. Pathology and clinical features.

    A. Ten percent are malignant. Incidence of malignancy increased in extraadrenal pheochromocytomas.

    B. Pheochromocytomas are predominantly sporadic; 10% occur in familial fashion, primarily MEN II A and B.

    C. Common presenting features include headache, palpitations, and hyperhydrosis.

    D. Although paroxysmal hypertension brought on by exercise, bending, urination, or anxiety brings pheochromocytoma to mind, the majority of patients show persistent hypertension.

    E. Diagnosis.

        1. Primarily through measurement of catecholamines in urine or serum.

        2. Use of imaging is for localization rather than diagnosis. Usual therapy is surgical removal.

    F. Radiographic and radionuclide imaging.

        1. Computed tomographic (CT) scanning is the primary technique for localization.

        2. Indications for radionuclide imaging with metaiodobenzylguanidine (MIBG) include:

a. Confirmation of equivocal CT scan.
b. Identification of extraadrenal sites.

Radiopharmaceutical

I. Metaiodobenzylguanidine is a synthesis of bretylium and guanethadine. These agents are known to localize in sympathetic tissue.
A. Dosimetry.
1. Usual dose—0.5 mCi.
2. Radiation dose is 100 rad/mCi to the adrenal medulla; total body is 0.1 rad/mCi.

Imaging Technique

I. Thyroid uptake of free radioiodine is blocked by the administration of saturated solution of potassium iodide (SSKI) beginning 24 hours before administration.
II. Material is injected IV and imaging is performed at 24, 48, and 72 hours. Whole-body imaging is performed.
III. Renal scanning is routinely used to outline kidneys and bladder. Computer substration is helpful.

Normal Study

I. Faint visualization of the normal adrenal medulla can be seen in approximately 16% of studies.
II. Liver uptake is uniformly seen being maximal at 24 hours.
III. Splenic uptake is normal because of the rich sympathetic enervation.
IV. Urinary bladder is seen since 60% of the injected material is excreted within the first 24 hours through the genitourinary (GU) tract.
V. Approximately 20% of studies show large bowel.
VI. The salivary glands are normally visualized, again, because of the rich sympathetic enervation.
VII. The heart is visualized due to sympathetics. Interestingly, an inverse linear relationship between plasma norepinephrine and intensity of heart uptake has been seen. The intensity of uptake is greater in patients who do not have a pheochromocytoma.

Abnormal Study

I. Abnormal uptake in the region of the adrenals is a primary finding.
II. Uptake in extra-adrenal sites, such as the organ of Zuckerkandl, are also abnormal. Note: pheochromocytomas in the bladder may be missed because of normal GU excretion. The renal scan can be helpful in this area.

Utility

I. Sensitivity for pheochromocytomas—85% to 90%.
II. Other uses.
   A. Other related tumors can be imaged and even treated with this material. These include neuroblastoma, carcinoid, and paragangliomas.

ADRENAL CORTICAL IMAGING (IODOMETHYL-19-NORCHOLESTEROL)

Anatomy

I. Adrenal cortex and medulla composed of entirely different tissues embryologically, histologically, and functionally.
II. Cortex constitutes 90% of gland volume. Divided into three histologic zones with different function.
   A. Zona glomerulosa—outermost zone produces aldosterone—the principal mineralocorticoid.
   B. Zona fasciculata—produces cortisol—principal glucocorticoid hormone.
   C. Zone reticularis—produces androgenic steriods—chiefly androstenedione.
III. Adrenal medulla secretes.
   A. Catecholamines.
      1. Epinephrine.
      2. Norepinephrine.
IV. Adrenal gland situated retroperitoneally superior and medial to upper pole of kidneys.
V. Right adrenal higher and more posterior than left; thus in normal adrenal scans, right gland will appear slightly hotter than left.
VI. Left adrenal slightly larger and crescentic; right, smaller and triangular.

Physiology

I. Secretory function of adrenal cortex is controlled primarily by anterior pituitary through ACTH.
II. Aldosterone secretion controlled by:
   A. Angiotensin II.
   B. Blood volume.
   C. Electrolyte concentration.
III. Cholesterol is stored in high concentration in adrenal cortex because it is principal metabolic precursor for the synthesis of adrenocorticosteroids including aldosterone. This forms basis for adrenal imaging.

Radiopharmaceutical

I. Iodomethyl-19-norcholesterol.
   A. As noted above, uptake dependent on fact that cholesterol is precursor in synthesis of adrenocorticosteroids.
   B. After IV injection, is bound to plasma low-density lipoproteins.
   C. Adrenal uptake increases with increased ACTH.
   D. Uptake occurs gradually over period of days.
   E. Adrenal-to-liver ratios—170:1.
   F. Adrenal-to-kidney ratios—300:1.
   G. Radiation dosimetry (rad/mCi).
      1. Adrenals—25.
      2. Ovaries—8.
      3. Testes—2.3.
      4. Total body—1.2.

Technique

I. Imaging.
   A. Patient pretreated with SSKI to prevent thyroid uptake of free radioiodine.
   B. Patient given 1 mCi per 1.7 sq m of body surface area (BSA) IV. Must be given slowly because rapid injections may cause histamine-release reaction.
   C. Imaging begins 48 hours after injection. Scan daily thereafter for 3 to 5 days.
   D. Posterior views obtained for 50,000 counts or 20 minutes.
II. Suppression test.
   A. Done for separation of aldosteronomas from hyperplasia.
   B. Patient given 4 mg of dexamethasone for 7 days before scanning.

Normal Scan

I. Bilateral symmetrical uptake. Note the right adrenal may appear slightly hotter than left posterior position.
II. On dexamethasone suppression, normally adrenals will not be seen for 5 days.
III. Uptakes may be performed similarly to thyroid uptakes. Normal is 0.07% to 0.26%.

Abnormal Studies

I. Cushing's syndrome.
   A. Resulting from excess of glucocorticosteroids—primarily cortisol.
   B. May be caused by:

1. Excessive ACTH secretions from:
   a. Pituitary.
   b. Ectopic sources.
2. ACTH—independent.
   a. Adrenal adenoma.
   b. Bilateral hyperplasia.
C. Clinical manifestations.
   1. Hypertension.
   2. Diabetes.
   3. Central obesity.
   4. Hirsutism.
   5. Plethora.
   6. Emotional lability.
   7. Osteoporosis.
   8. Cutaneous striae.
D. Laboratory findings.
   1. Elevated plasma cortisol.
   2. Absence of normal diurnal variation of cortisol.
   3. High doses of dexamethasone suppress pituitary adenomas producing ACTH.
   4. Increase urinary glucocorticoid metabolites after metapyrone in ACTH-dependent disease.
E. Scan findings.
   1. Increased symmetrical uptake—bilateral hyperplasia.
      a. Note that ACTH-independent tumors of adrenal cortex and ectopic ACTH produce higher uptakes than pituitary-dependent ACTH Cushing's syndrome.
F. Asymmetrical uptake.
   1. Asymmetric hyperplasia.
   2. Combination hyperplasia/adenoma.
G. Unilateral uptake—adenoma.
H. No uptake—carcinoma.
I. Accuracy—90%.
II. Aldosteronism.
A. Aldosterone does not suppress ACTH production. Aldosteronoma results in asymmetrical appearance rather than unilateral visualization. Unfortunately, asymmetry cannot be distinguished from asymmetrical hyperplasia.
B. Dexamethasone suppression test useful in differentiation.
   1. Hyperplasia—symmetrical uptake visualized before 5 days.
C. Adenoma—early visualization with absent or poor visualization in opposite adrenal.
D. Normal—no visualization for 5 days.

E. Sensitivity and accuracy—90%. Note that diuretics stimulate renin and can increase adrenal uptake of cholesterol and radioiodinated cholesterol, mimicking bilateral hyperplasia. Note also, early uptake has been described in oral contraceptives, again resulting from increased plasma renin.

III. Low-renin hypertension.

A. When scanned with adrenal corticol suppression, full range of suppression-scan images found, as in aldosteronism.

IV. Androgen excess.

A. Usually excess androgens causing virilism secondary to ovarian production; however, can occur from adrenals. Because androgen production does not affect release of ACTH, suppression scanning necessary.

B. Bilateral early visualization—bilateral hyperplasia.

C. Unilateral visualization—adrenal adenoma.

D. Bilateral visualization greater than 5 days—normal response.

E. Note that early visualization has been observed in some patients taking oral contraceptives.

SUGGESTED READINGS

Beierwaltes WH: Treatment of hyperthyroidism with iodine-131. *Semin Nucl Med* 1978; 8:95-103.

Beierwaltes WH: Treatment of thyroid carcinoma with radioactive iodine. *Semin Nucl Med* 1978; 8:79-93.

Beierwaltes WH, Nishiyama RH, Thompson NW, et al: Survival time and "cure" in papillary and follicular thyroid carcinoma with distant metastases: Statistics following University of Michigan therapy. *J Nucl Med* 1982; 23:561-568.

Beierwaltes WH, Rabbani R, Dmuchowski C, et al: Analysis of "ablation of thyroid remnants" with I-131 in 511 patients from 1947-1984: Experience at University of Michigan. *J Nucl Med* 1984; 25:1287-1293.

Bravo EL, Gifford RW: Pheochromocytoma: Diagnosis, localization and management. *New Engl J Med* 1984; 311:1296-1302.

Echenique RL, Kasi L, Haynie TP, et al: Critical evaluation of serum thyroglobulin levels and I-131 scans in post-therapy patients with differentiated thyroid carcinoma: Concise communication. *J Nucl Med* 1982; 23:235-240.

Favus MJ, Schneider AB, Stachura ME, et al: Thyroid cancer occurring as a late consequence of head-and-neck irradiation: evaluation of 1056 patients. *New Engl J Med* 1976; 294:1019-1025.

Ferlin G, Borsato N, Camerani M, et al: New perspectives in localizing enlarged parathyroids by technetium-thallium subtraction scan. *J Nucl Med* 1983; 24:438-441.

Freitas JE, Gross MD, Ripley S, et al: Radio-nuclide diagnosis and therapy of thyroid cancer: Current status report. *Semin Nucl Med* 1985; 15:106-130.

Guerra UP, Pizzocaro C, Terzi A, et al: New tracers for imaging medullary thyroid carcinoma. *Nucl Med Commun* 1989; 10:285-295.

Hubert JP, Kiernan PD, Beahrs OH, et al: Occult papillary carcinoma of the thyroid. *Arch Surg* 115:394-398.

Hurley JR, Becker DV: Use of radioiodine in the management of thyroid cancer. In Freeman LM, Weissman HS (eds): *Nuclear medicine annual 1983.* New York, Raven, pp 329-382.

Keyes JW, Thrall JH, Carey JE: Technical considerations in in vivo thyroid studies. *Semin Nucl Med* 1978; 8:43-57.

Kimmig B, Brandeis WE, Eisenhut M, et al: Scintigraphy of a neuroblastoma with I-131 meta-iodobenzylguanidine. *J Nucl Med* 1984; 25:773-774.

Kuni CC, Klingensmith WC: Failure of low doses of ^{131}I to ablate residual thyroid tissue following surgery for thyroid cancer. *Radiology* 1980; 137:773-775.

MacFarlane SD, Hanelin LG, Taft DA, et al: Localization of abnormal parathyroid glands using thallium-201. *Am J Surg* 1984; 148:7-13.

Mazzaferri EL: Papillary and follicular thyroid cancer: A selective approach to diagnosis and treatment. *Ann Rev Med* 1981; 32:73-91.

McDermott MT, Kidd GS, Dodson LE, et al. Radioiodine-induced thyroid storm. *Am J Med* 1983; 74:353-359.

McEwan AJ, Shapiro B, Sisson JC, et al: Radioiodobenzylguanidine for the scintigraphic location and therapy of adrenergic tumors. *Semin Nucl Med* 1985; 15:132-153.

O'Doherty MJ, Kettle AG, Wells P, et al: Parathyroid imaging with ^{99m}Tc sestamibi: Preoperative localization and tissue uptake studies. *J Nucl Med* 1992; 33:313-318.

Parisi MT, Greene MK, Dykes TM, et al: Efficacy of metaiodobenzylguanidine as a scintigraphic agent for detection of neuroblastoma. *Investig Radiol* 1992; 27:768-773.

Pinsky S, Ryo UY: Thyroid imaging: A current status report. In Freeman LM, Weissman HS (eds): *Nuclear medicine annual 1981.* New York, Raven, pp 157-193.

Potchen EJ: Parathyroid imaging: Current status and future prospects. *J Nucl Med* 1992; 33:1807-1809.

Robertson JS, Gorman CA: Gonadal radiation dose and its genetic significance in radiation therapy of hyperthyroidism. *J Nucl Med* 1976; 17:826-835.

Samaan NA, Schultz PN, Hickey RC, et al: Results of various treatment modalities of well-differentiated thyroid carcinoma: A retrospective review of 1599 patients. *J Clin Endocrin Metab* 1992; 75:714-720.

Sarkar SD, Beierwaltes WH, Gill SP, et al: Subsequent fertility and birth histories of children and adolescents treated with ^{131}I for thyroid cancer. *J Nucl Med* 1976; 17:460-464.

Shapiro B, Copp JE, Sisson JC, et al: Iodine-131 metaiodobenzyl-guanidine for the locating of suspected pheochromocytoma: Experience in 400 cases. *J Nucl Med* 1985; 26:576-585.

Sisson JC, Frager MS, Valk TW, et al: Scintigraphic localization of pheochromocytoma. *New Engl J Med* 1981; 305:11-17.

Sridama V, McCormick M, Kaplan EL, et al: Long-term followup study of compensated low dose ^{131}I therapy for Graves' disease. *New Engl J Med* 1984; 311:426-432.

Taillefer R, Boucher Y, Potvin C, et al: Detection and localization of parathyroid adenomas in patients with hyperparathyroidism using single radionuclide imaging procedure with ^{99m}Tc-sestamibi (double-phase study). *J Nucl Med* 1992; 33:1801-1807.

Winzelberg GG, Hydovitz JD, O'Hara KR, et al: Parathyroid adenomas evaluated by Tl-201/Tc-99m pertechnetate subtraction scintigraphy and high-resolution ultrasonography. *Radiology* 1985; 155:231-235.

Young RL, Nusynowitz ML: Treatment of benign thyroid disease. *Semin Nucl Med* 1979; 9:85-93.

2

Central Nervous System Imaging

CENTRAL NERVOUS SYSTEM
Anatomy

I. Blood supply.
    A. Arterial.
        1. Carotid and vertebral basilar systems.
            a. Communication of carotid and basilar systems through circle of Willis—posterior and anterior communicating arteries.
        2. Cerebral hemispheres.
            a. Supplied by:
                (1) Anterior cerebral arteries—branch of internal carotid.
                (2) Middle cerebral artery—branch of internal carotid.
                (3) Posterior cerebral artery—branch of the basilar artery.
            b. Distribution of flow to the cerebrum allows vascular lesions to be identified (Figure 2-1).
            c. The area representing boundaries of vessel's vascular supply is called the watershed.
        3. Cerebellum and brain stem.
            a. Supplied by the basilar artery.
    B. Venous drainage
        1. Through venous sinuses.
            a. The flow pattern is through sagittal sinus (runs anterior-posteriorly in falx cerebri) and transverse sinuses (run laterally-medially in tentorium cerebelli); these meet at torcular hermophilae; blood proceeds through to the transverse sinus, then to the sigmoid sinus, and into the jugular vein.

II. Cerebrospinal fluid (CSF).
    A. Forms a large space in each hemisphere.
    B. CSF drains from lateral ventricles through foramen of Monroe to midline third ventricle through aqueduct of Sylvius, to fourth ventricle. CSF leaves fourth ventricle through foramina of Luschka and Magendie entering cisterna magna.

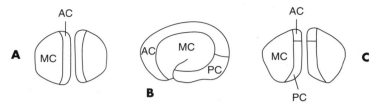

Fig. 2-1 Vascular distribution on, **A**, anterior, **B**, lateral, and, **C**, posterior brain scan views. *AC*, anterior cerebral; *MC*, middle cerebral; *PC*, posterior cerebral.

Physiology

I. Blood-brain barrier prevents most materials from being transported from blood into neural tissues. Has both anatomic and physiologic basis.
   A. Brain capillaries, unlike other capillaries, have a continuous basement membrane and closed endothelial clefts (tight junctions) preventing movement of large molecular-weight proteins.
   B. Close approximation of astrocyte foot processes, restricts entry of material.
   C. Passive diffusion, pore filtration, and pinocytosis normally do not occur.
   D. Instead, movement of substances across capillaries is by active transport.
   E. Blood-brain barrier normally prevents routine radiopharmaceuticals from entering brain. Diseases that result in radiopharmaceutical uptake cause breakdown of the blood-brain barrier, allowing radiopharmaceuticals to cross. In tumors, uptake results from:
      1. Blood-brain barrier breakdown.
      2. Increased vascularity.
      3. Abnormal permeability.
      4. Pinocytosis.
      5. Increased size of extracellular space.
      6. Cerebral edema.
      7. Direct intracellular uptake.

Conventional Planar Radiopharmaceuticals

I. Technetium 99m pertechnetate.
   A. Most commonly used conventional planar brain scanning agent.
   B. Following IV injection, loosely bound to albumin.
   C. Because of slow blood clearance, delayed imaging 3 to 4 hours after injection is required.
   D. Pertechnetate normally concentrated by choroid plexus. Potassium

Table 2-1   Conventional Planar Brain Scanning Agents

Radiopharmaceutical	Dose (mCi)	Imaging Delay (Hr)
^{99m}Tc Pertechnetate*	10-20	2-4
^{99m}Tc DTPA	15-20	1-3
^{99m}Tc glucohepatonate	15-20	1-2

*Premedicate with 200 mg of potassium perchlorate.

      perchlorate given orally to block uptake. Perchlorate has little effect on salivary and oral uptake of pertechnetate, however.

II. Technetium diethylenetriamine pentaacetic acid (DTPA) and gluco-heptonate.

  A. These renal agents have enhanced renal excretion and diminished background activity. Allows earlier imaging and, theoretically, increased sensitivity.

  B. These agents are not normally concentrated in the choroid plexus; perchlorate pretreatment unnecessary.

  C. Increased sensitivity over pertechnetate is seen in lesions with poor uptake.

    1. Acute infarcts.

    2. Well-differentiated gliomas.

    3. Tumors near base of brain.

  D. Glucoheptonate slightly superior to DTPA.

Conventional Planar Technique

  I. Radionuclide angiogram.

    A. Bolus injection in antecubital vein (see Table 2-1 for dose). Two-second analogue and 0.5 frames/second computer images obtained for 60 seconds.

  II. Immediate blood pool images in anterior, lateral, posterior projections.

  III. Delayed images.

    A. Delay dependent on radiopharmaceutical used (see Table 2-1).

    B. Anterior, both laterals, posteriors routinely. Vertex and posterior fossa views with head in flexion, as needed.

    C. One million count anterior view with pertechnetate. Fewer counts for others. Other views obtained for time of anterior view.

Normal Studies

  I. Flow study—anterior view.

    A. Three phases.

      1. Arterial phase.

a. Activity in subclavian vessels, symmetric common carotid, symmetric middle cerebral arteries laterally and anterior cerebral arteries medially.

b. Anterior cerebrals superimposed on one another, appear as single vessel.

2. Capillary phase.

a. Symmetric diffuse activity in both cerebral hemispheres.

3. Venous phase.

a. Sagittal sinus and jugular vessels visualized. Note jugular venous drainage can be asymmetric.

II. Flow study—posterior view.

A. Same three phases showing symmetric vertebral arteries.

III. Flow study—vertex view.

A. Major vessels not well seen.

B. Capillary phases of anterior, middle and posterior cerebral arteries can all be evaluated on this one view, however.

C. Computer analysis of hemispheric regions can be helpful in differentiating subtle differences in perfusion.

IV. Blood pool images—significant soft-tissue and venous sinus activity.

V. Delayed static views.

1. Anterior.

a. Superior rim of activity that widens in the lower margins as a result of scalp, skull, meninges, and temporalis muscle activity.

b. Sagittal sinus in midline extending downward variable distance.

c. Inferiorly, orbits appear above diffuse face and skull base activity. Cerebral cortex normally devoid of activity.

2. Lateral.

a. Mirror images.

b. Outer line of activity because of scalp/skull.

c. Inner line—sagittal sinus.

d. Sagittal sinus thins anteriorly, thickens posteriorly.

e. Inferiorly, facial activity.

f. Ear and temporalis muscle may be seen.

3. Posterior.

a. Rim of activity, thickens in lower margins because of sigmoid sinuses.

b. Inferiorly, sagittal and transverse sinuses.

c. Occasionally, occipital sinus seen.

d. Common variant—small or absent left transverse sinus.

4. Vertex view.

a. Superior sagittal sinus divides brain into left and right hemispheres. Anteriorly, increased activity due to salivary glands, activity in nasopharynx, and increased vascularity. Laterally, parotid activity seen with pertechnetate.

Abnormal Conventional Planar Studies

I. Flow study.
  A. Asymmetry of absence of flow most common abnormality.
  B. Increased flow less commonly seen.
II. Blood pools.
  A. Increased activity that may either fade or increase with time, helpful in differentiating vascular lesions from tumor.
III. Delayed imaging.
  A. Increased uptake in the regions of the cortex.
IV. Specific disease processes in which conventional planar scan is used.
  A. Brain death.
    1. Background.
      a. Abnormal radionuclide brain scan is a commonly accepted criterion for brain death. Can be performed at bedside. Primary use of conventional brain scan at present.
    2. Findings.
      a. Angiogram.
        (1) Normal carotid activity without anterior or middle cerebral perfusion on anterior view; external flow expected; tourniquet can be used to prevent this, if desired.
        (2) Immediate images.
          (a) No evidence of sinus uptake.
        (3) Delayed statics.
          (a) No evidence of dural sinus.
          (b) Occasionally, sagittal or transverse sinus faintly seen. May be caused by collateral circulation from scalp or drainage through basilar system with reflux into sinuses. Still considered brain dead.
          (c) In children, visualization of sutures also considered a sign of brain death. Seen because of diminished background activity without cerebral perfusion.
    3. Scan can be repeated in 8 hours if first study is negative.
  B. Inflammatory disease.
    1. Herpex simplex.
      a. Background.
        (1) Most common cause of sporadic encephalitis in United States. Insidious onset.
        (2) Symptoms—headache, lethargy, fever, followed by confusion, disorientation, seizure, and coma.

    b. Sensitivity—50% to 85%. Radionuclide examination may become positive earlier than computed tomography (CT).

    c. Findings.

        (1) Most specific—bilateral hyperfusion with bilateral temporal increased activity on delayed images.

        (2) Other patterns:

            (a) Unilateral hyperfusion with unilateral temporal-frontal uptake.

            (b) Decreased flow secondary to necrosis.

        (3) Differential diagnosis of pattern includes:

            (a) Cerebritis.

            (b) Abscess.

            (c) Cerebral infarction with luxury perfusion.

            (d) Vascular tumor.

  2. Brain abscess/cerebritis.

    a. Background.

        (1) Cause—sepsis or contiguous spread.

        (2) Frequently multiple.

        (3) Symptoms—fever or neurologic dysfunction.

    b. Sensitivity—90%. At cerebritis stage radionuclide may be more sensitive than CT.

    c. Findings.

        (1) Focally increased flow.

        (2) Increased uptake on statics, approximately 50% showing doughnut sign.

        (3) Differential diagnosis of doughnut sign.

            (a) Metastasis.

            (b) Glioblastoma.

            (c) Stroke.

            (d) Hematoma.

            (e) Radiation necrosis.

V. Diseases sometimes seen when doing scans for reasons above. Scan no longer used for primary diagnosis of diseases discussed below.

A. Cerebrovascular disease.

  1. Stroke/atherosclerotic disease.

    a. Background.

        (1) Third most common cause of death.

        (2) Strokes due to thrombosis, hemorrhage, or embolism.

        (3) Three fourths of all thromboses involve internal carotid/middle cerebral artery.

        (4) Transient ischemic attacks (TIAs) often precursor to stroke.

    b. Sensitivity of flow study—varies with degree of stenosis.

(1) >80% stenosis—80% sensitivity.

(2) 50% stenosis—50% sensitivity.

(3) <50% stenosis—10% or less sensitivity.

(4) Since asymmetry is a primary finding, lower sensitivity for bilateral disease.

(5) Sensitivity of delayed images for stroke varies with timing.

    (a) Most sensitive 3 to 4 weeks after event.

    (b) <25% sensitivity in first week.

(6) Hemorrhagic strokes more likely to be positive than ischemic.

(7) Internal capsule, basal ganglia, brainstem infarcts usually missed because of their small size.

(8) Completed cerebral infarction—50% to 80% show perfusion asymmetry.

(9) False-positive flow studies in 20% of patients with nonfocal neurologic disease, 15% of normals in advanced age group.

(10) Radionuclide angiogram most sensitive for occlusion carotid or proximal middle cerebral artery.

(11) Vertebrobasilar lesions missed 80% of time.

(12) TIAs.

    (a) Radionuclide detects approximately one half with unilateral stenosis, 29% with bilateral stenosis, 11% with plaques and ulcerations.

c. Findings.

  (1) Atherosclerosis without stroke.

    (a) Asymmetric decreased flow.

    (b) Bilateral decreased flow more difficult to evaluate. Congestive heart failure and slow circulation times can give false-positive appearance of bilateral disease.

    (c) Differential diagnosis of hypoperfusion:

      (i) Atherosclerotic stroke.

      (ii) Large subdural hematoma.

      (iii) Other avascular masses.

  (2) Stroke.

    (a) Cerebral angiogram.

      (i) Asymmetric decreased flow with internal carotid occlusion.

      (ii) Hot nose because of increased external carotid flow may be present with internal carotid occlusion.

      (iii) Flip-flop sign.

          a Arterial phase—decreased involved side, normal opposite side. Later phases—increased involved side, decreased normal side. Due to collateral circulation to involved area with delayed entry.

      (iv) Luxury perfusion—occasional increased flow with stroke—luxury perfusion resulting from reactive hyperemia.

   (b) Static images.
      (i) Increased uptake.
      (ii) Characteristically flame-shaped.
      (iii) Occurs in region of flow abnormality.

   (c) Hemorrhagic stroke.
      (i) Statics normal early.
      (ii) One-fourth positive in first week, fade by 6 to 8 weeks.
      (iii) Hemorrhagic more commonly seen in the first week than ischemic.

B. Arteriovenous malformations (AVMs).
  1. Background—congenital or acquired. May be single or multiple.
  2. Signs and symptoms—seizures or evidence of intracranial bleeding.
  3. Sensitivity—80% to 95%, those missed usually less than 1.5 cm.
  4. Findings:
    a. Radiounuclide angiogram
      (1) Early blush during arterial phase that fades during venous phase.
      (2) Early appearance of dural sinuses also seen.
    b. Immediate images.
      (1) Increased blood pool.
      (2) Enlarged seeding/draining vessels.
    c. Static images.
      (1) Normal—activity fading with time differentiates AVM from vascular tumor.

C. Aneurysms.
    a. Background—most common cause of subarachnoid hemorrhage.
    b. Sensitivity—rarely detected unless large.
    c. Findings.
      (1) Focal area of increased flow on flow study.
      (2) If it has bled, induced vascular spasm may be detected as decreased perfusion.

D. Tumors.
  1. General.
    a. Sensitivity—CT at least 10% more sensitive for detection (95% vs 85%). Depends on type and location of tumor.
    b. Tumor type.
      (1) Best—radionuclides.
        (a) Glioblastoma multiforme.
        (b) Meningioma.
        (c) Some metastatic tumors.
      (2) Worst—radionuclides.
        (a) Low-grade astrocytomas.
        (b) Pinealoma.
        (c) Cystic lesions.
        (d) Some metastatic lesions.
    c. Location—poorest:
      (1) Base of brain.
      (2) Adjacent to vascular structures.
    d. Size—<1 cm, usually missed unless associated with significant reactive edema.
  2. Gliomas.
    a. Background.
      (1) Glial tumors most common tumor type in both adults and children.
        (a) One half of all tumors in adults are gliomas.
        (b) Three fourths in pediatrics are gliomas.
      (2) Adults—glioblastoma multiforme in cerebral hemisphere is most common.
      (3) Children—cystic astrocytoma and infratentorial medulloblastoma is most common.
    b. Findings.
      (1) Glioblastoma multiforme.
        (a) Delayed images.
          (i) Significant increased uptake, due to neovascularity.
        (b) If large area of necrosis present, doughnut pattern seen. Necrosis occurs because of rapid growth, outgrows blood supply.
        (c) Distribution of activity may be irregular; tumor may cross arterial blood supply boundaries. May extend across midline into opposite hemisphere (butterfly glioma).
      (2) Low-grade astrocytomas.

        (a) Mild focal uptake.

        (b) Have little neovascularity and cause little breakdown of blood-brain barrier.

3. Meningioma.

  a. Background.

    (1) Slow-growing, highly vascular tumor arising from meninges in regions of arachnoid granulations.

    (2) More common in women.

    (3) Can occur following trauma.

  b. Sensitivity.

    (1) Tumor for which radionuclides have highest sensitivity, >90%.

  c. Findings.

    (1) Flow study—hypervascular arteriovenous phases.

    (2) Immediates—increased uptake.

    (3) Delayed—significant increased uptake that increases with time compared with immediates. Activity usually located sagittal, parasagittal, or along sphenoid wings.

4. Metastases.

  a. Background.

    (1) Accounts for one fourth of brain tumors.

    (2) Most common primary:

      (a) Lung.

      (b) Breast.

      (c) Kidney.

      (d) Melanomas.

    (3) Most common symptom—headache.

  b. Sensitivity.

    (1) Approximately 80%.

    (2) National Cancer Institute study found almost no cases in which radionuclide study was positive in face of negative CT scan.

    (3) Steroid therapy decreases sensitivity.

  c. Findings.

    (1) Cerebral angiogram.

      (a) Usually normal. With large/hypervascular tumors, increased activity seen. Occasionally, displacement of vessels seen.

      (b) Delayed images—increased uptake. Only distinguishing characteristic of metastatic tumors is multiplicity. Majority of metastases are multiple, supratentorial, and frequently in middle cerebral artery (MCA) distribution. Note degree of uptake may vary between sites because of biologic differences and degree of reactive edema.

E. Trauma.
  1. Subdural hematomas.
    a. Background.
      (1) Caused by rupture of veins bridging cerebral hemi-spheres entering dural sinuses.
    b. Sensitivity.
      (1) Flow study: detects 85% to 90% of subdurals. Smaller subdurals (axis displacement <3.6 cm) missed.
      (2) Static images: sensitivity depends on timing. Normal first week, chronic subdurals best seen at 2 weeks.
    c. Findings.
      (1) Cerebral angiogram.
        (a) Medial displacement of cerebral hemisphere, which persists through arteriovenous phases.
        (b) Occasional patients show increased activity, pre-sumably from rapid leakage across damaged blood-brain barrier or crowding of vessels.
      (2) Static images.
        (a) Usually negative in acute subdurals.
        (b) 7 to 10 days peripheral crescent of activity resulting from:
          (i) Edema.
          (ii) New vessel formation.
          (iii) Other factors.
          (iv) Note crescent sign not specific for subdural. May be seen in scalp contusions, lacerations, hematomas, skull fractures, etc.
  2. Contusion.
    a. Background.
      (1) Most frequently in temporal lobe—often bilateral because of contracoup injury.
    b. Sensitivity—usually missed in first week.
    c. Findings.
      (1) Radionuclide angiogram.
        (a) Normal differentiates from subdural.
      (2) Static images.
        (a) Increased uptake.

Functional (SPECT) Radiopharmaceuticals

I. Conventional brain imaging agents enter the brain *only* if a break-down of the blood-brain barrier (BBB) occurs. This causes focal increased uptake in areas where structural abnormalities (e.g., abscess or tumor) are present. The new functional SPECT agents, on the other hand, are able to cross the intact BBB. Their uptake is correlated with regional cerebral blood flow, local metabolism, or receptor levels.

II. Brain perfusion agents—minimum criteria for agents to measure regional cerebral blood flow:
 A. Pass through intact BBB.
 B. High first-pass extraction.
 C. Prolonged retention in brain (at least 30 to 60 minutes to allow completion of SPECT imaging).
 D. No significant redistribution before or during imaging.
 E. Little or no metabolism or biologic effects.

III. IMP-N-isopropyl ^{123}I p-iodoamphetamine.
 A. Neutral, lipid soluble, aromatic monoamine originally developed as a neural transmitter analog. Distribution reflects regional cerebral blood flow.
 B. Uptake in brain because of high lipid solubility; readily crosses the intact BBB. First-pass extraction is 85% to 95%.
 C. Total activity constant for 20 to 60 minutes after injection. Most likely explanation for trapping of IMP is pH change. Intracellular space of brain has a lower pH, causing the agent to lose its lipophilicity. Other mechanisms likely contribute, as well.
 D. Seven percent of injected dose enters brain; other organs with high uptake include liver and lung.
 E. Note: image quality varies by how ^{123}I was produced in cyclotron.
  1. Direct method — (^{124}Te) (p, 2n) > ^{123}I contaminated with 2% to 4% ^{124}I. 603-KeV photons degrade image. A 100-hour half-life increases radiation dose.
  2. Indirect method.
   a. ^{127}I^{p,5n} Y Xe ^{123}I.
   b. ^{123}I contaminated with ^{125}I, which is much less of a problem.
 F. Redistribution can occur in ischemia, similar to that seen in the heart with ^{201}Tl.
 G. Absorbed radiation dose—N-isopropyl-^{123}I p-iodoamphetamine.

Target Organ	Rad/6 mCi
Brain	0.58
Retina	4.4
Lens	0.76
Lung	1.4
Liver	1.3
Kidneys	0.42

Bladder	2.2
Testes	0.38
Ovaries	0.47
Total body	0.46

H. HIPDM is a diamine, similar in biodistribution to IMP.

IV. HMPAO - hexamethylpropyleneamine oxime—d,l isomer shows brain retention; mesoisomer shows little in vivo brain retention.

A. Liquid soluble passes through intact BBB.

B. High first-pass extraction.

C. Retention similar to IMP. Trapped in brain by reaction with intracellular glutathione; converts it to a nonlipophilic moiety.

D. No redistribution occurs.

E. No significant biologic effects.

F. Estimated absorbed radiation dose — ^{99m}Tc HMPAO.

Target Organ	Rad/20 mCi
Lacrymal glands	5.16
Gallbladder wall	3.80
Kidney	2.60
Thyroid	1.00
Upper large intestine wall	1.58
Liver	1.08
Small intestine wall	0.88
Lower large intestine wall	1.08
Urinary bladder wall	0.94
Brain	0.52
Ovaries	0.46
Testes	0.14
Whole body	0.26

Technique

I. IMP.

A. Patient is placed in a quiet room.

B. Patient is injected with 5 mCi intravenously; imaging begins 15 minutes later.

C. High-resolution collimator of medium energy (because of contamination by ^{124}I) used on single-, dual-, and triple-headed SPECT camera.

D. Rotation of 360 degrees, 64 stops, 40 seconds/stop.

II. HMPAO.

A. Patient is placed in quiet room with eyes closed.

B. Patient is injected with 25 mCi intravenously; imaging begins 10 minutes later.

C. High-resolution technetium collimator used.

D. SPECT acquisition performed with 64 × 64 matrix.

1. Single-head 360-degree rotation, 128 stops, 15 seconds/stop.
2. Triple-headed system: 1.3 hardware zoom; 120 stops, 20 seconds/stop.

Normal Scan

I. Symmetric uptake, predominantly in gray matter of brain.
II. Note: Small areas of decreased activity are frequently seen around cortex in each tomographic slice.

Abnormal Scan

I. Areas of increased or decreased activity.
II. Specific disease processes.
   A. Cerebrovascular disease.
     1. Stroke.
       a. Findings.
         (1) Decreased focal uptake.
         (2) Increased uptake occasionally seen, more commonly with HMPAO, due to luxury perfusion. Loss of autoregulation of cerebral blood flow in the peri-infarct region results in hyperemia. Effect is transient and not seen on scans performed after the acute event.
         (3) Crossed cerebellar diaschisis also sometimes occurs. Cerebellar flow and metabolism contralateral to area of infarction are diminished, probably caused by disruption of corticopontine neuronal connections. Decreased uptake in the contralateral cerebellar hemisphere is seen.
         (4) Overall size of infarct is usually larger on SPECT than CT or MRI. This is due to both surrounding ischemia identified with SPECT blood flow agents and autoregulation of blood flow, which causes decreased regional cerebral blood flow to areas of the brain dependent on the damaged portion for neuronal activity.
       b. Sensitivity and specificity.
         (1) Overall sensitivity for gray matter infarcts is similar to CT; however, because of predominantly gray matter uptake and poorer spatial resolution, most lacunar and white matter infarctions are missed. Nonetheless, SPECT agents can demonstrate acute strokes earlier than CT.
       c. Uses:
         (1) Diagnosis of stroke in selected patients. CT/MR is still recommended in the majority of patients, since these modalities have high sensitivity and specificity and

allow differentiation of hemorrhagic vs. ischemic infarct.

(2) To identify ischemia *before* an infarct develops. This allows interventions to be applied in the hope of preventing permanent damage.

(a) An IMP scan can be performed immediately and at 4 hours. Patients who show redistribution have cerebral tissue at risk and will benefit the most from interventions.

(3) Prognosis.

(a) Size and location of defect is of *some* utility (although very imperfect) for predicting outcome of a stroke.

(b) Patients demonstrating IMP redistribution have a better clinical prognosis than patients not showing the sign.

(4) Subarachnoid hemorrhage.

(a) A third of patients develop arterial vasospasm.

(b) Scan can detect this. Information useful for timing interventions and measuring effectiveness of treatment.

2. Vascular disease.

a. TIAs can show initial defect at time of symptoms that fills-in on delayed imaging. Between attacks, the scan is normal.

b. Preoperative and postoperative carotid endarterectomy scans can be performed to document success (controversial).

c. Acetazolamide (diamox) test.

(1) Background.

(a) Acetazolamide is a carbonic anhydrase inhibitor. By changing cerebral levels of CO_2 (or via other mechanisms), a dose-dependent increase in cerebral blood flow X 2 occurs.

(b) Examination is similar to dipyridamole thallium study. It is done to test cerebrovascular hemodynamic reserve. Acetazolamide induces cerebrovascular vasodilatation. Since ischemic areas have already maximally vasodilated in response to ischemia, they have decreased perfusion reserve and therefore cannot respond. Normal areas increase blood flow $\times$ 2. This produces heterogeneity on scan that can be used to identify cerebrovascular disease that may infarct. Surgery or other interventions may be instituted immediately in hope of preventing a future CVA.

   (2) Technique.

      (a) 1 g of acetazolamide is injected IV over 2 minutes.

      (b) 25 minutes later, HMPAO is injected.

      (c) 15 to 25 minutes after injection, cerebral SPECT is performed.

      (d) A second "rest" study is performed before or after the pharmacologic examination. This is used to differentiate ischemia from infarct (as in a thallium cardiac study).

   (3) Findings.

      (a) Decreased uptake relative to remainder of brain in cerebral areas with vascular disease.

  d. Balloon occlusion.

   (1) Background.

      (a) SPECT HMPAO performed in cases of internal carotid aneurysm or cerebral tumor, in which occlusion or sacrifice of the internal carotid artery may be necessary. Circle of Willis provides collateral circulation but is completely intact in only 21% of individuals. HMPAO balloon occlusion study allows surgeon to predict outcome of loss of internal carotid artery on one side (i.e., determine if a stroke will result).

      (b) Scan necessary since 5% to 20% of patients *without* clinical symptoms during balloon occlusion of the internal carotid artery go on to infarct if the vessel is permanently occluded.

   (2) Technique.

      (a) Internal carotid artery is occluded with a balloon catheter during carotid angiogram.

      (b) 10 to 15 minutes into occlusion, 20 mCi of ^{99m}Tc HMPAO is injected.

      (c) Occlusion maintained (unless neurologic symptoms develop) for additional 15 to 20 minutes (30 minutes total occlusion).

      (d) SPECT study performed.

   (3) Findings.

      (a) Decreased flow on side with occlusion means region is in jeopardy if internal carotid artery is occluded or hypoperfusion occurs during surgery.

e. Matas test—similar to above but performed with manual occlusion of internal carotid artery.

B. Brain death.
  1. Using HMPAO has several potential advantages over using free pertechnetate in a radionuclide angiogram.
     a. A radionuclide angiogram can still be performed.
     b. The diagnosis is not completely dependent on the quality of the bolus. If a technical problem occurs or if the patient is in cardiac failure and has a slow circulation time, the uptake (or lack thereof) on delayed images can be used to make (or refute) the diagnosis of brain death. Note: A good-quality bolus is often difficult to achieve in children.
     c. The diagnosis of brain death is not solely dependent on flow measurement.
        (1) HMPAO uptake is dependent on *viable* tissue allowing the lipophilic agent to cross the blood-brain barrier and become trapped.
     d. The cerebellum can also be evaluated. Only anterior circulation is evaluated on radionuclide angiograms. Some patients may show absent supratentorial flow but intact cerebellar flow.
  2. Disadvantages.
     a. If patient's brain is shown to be viable, performing a repeat study a few hours later is more difficult.
     b. More expensive.
  3. Technique:
     a. Patient is injected with 20 mCi of ^{99m}Tc HMPAO intravenously.
        (1) Must perform chromatography and document that >90% of the HMPAO is in the lipophilic form.
        (2) Must inject drug within 30 minutes of preparation.
     b. A standard radionuclide angiogram is performed.
     c. Anterior and both lateral planar images (5 minutes imaging time each) are obtained 5 to 15 minutes after injection.
     d. An image over the chest and abdomen is also performed (as part of pharmaceutical quality control).
     e. SPECT is performed in questionable cases.
  4. Interpretation.
     a. No uptake in the cerebrum or cerebellum.
     b. No evidence of excessive thyroid or salivary uptake (indicates tag quality is good, no free pertechnetate).
     c. Normal chest/abdominal biodistribution (no stomach activity, which would indicate a poor tag). Lungs (lower two-thirds), liver, kidney, and bladder are normally seen.

C. Epilepsy.
1. Background.
   a. In the United States, 800,000 persons have partial seizures that do not generalize to major motor seizures or become complex. Approximately 20% of these patients fail medical treatment. If surgery is contemplated, exact localization is needed.
   b. EEG is valuable in diagnosing seizure disorders, but does not give detailed information about the location of the seizure focus.
   c. CT demonstrates an anatomic abnormality in only 10% to 40% of patients.
   d. SPECT can be useful in localizing seizure focus.
2. Technique.
   a. Radiopharmaceutical.
      (1) IMP is often preferable because it can be kept at bedside and injected when patient spontaneously has a seizure.
      (2) HMPAO must be used within 30 minutes of preparation; therefore, it is best to attempt to induce seizures if this material is used.
   b. During seizure, IMP or HMPAO is injected.
   c. SPECT imaging is performed.
3. Findings:
   a. Increased uptake in seizure focus with ictal scan.
   b. Interictal studies may show decreased activity in seizure focus.
   c. Size and location more accurate with ictal studies or post-ictal scan in first 5 minutes.
   d. As seizure activity generalizes, uptake of SPECT agents may give erroneous location information.
4. Sensitivity and specificity.
   a. As noted above, higher with ictal scans.
   b. Sensitivity.
      (1) SPECT alone—60% to 70%.
      (2) Combined EEG and SPECT—increases yield.
5. SPECT scans also sometimes used to differentiate seizures from pseudoseizures.
   a. Ictal injection shows marked focal uptake in true seizures and normal or less marked uptake with pseudoseizures.
   b. Note: Voluntary movement increases brain activation; therefore, some increased uptake can be present with pseudoseizures. This can make differentiation from true seizures difficult if increased uptake is present.

D. Dementia.
   1. Background.
      a. Alzheimer's disease is a chronic, progressive, degenerative disease of the CNS that causes dementia. Memory impairment, language difficulties and loss of cognitive capabilities occur.
        (1) Disease affects 2 million Americans over age 50.
        (2) Misdiagnoses are made in 10% to 30%.
        (3) No clinical signs or laboratory tests are pathognomonic.
        (4) CT and MR show no structural changes (although they can be helpful in excluding other causes of dementia such as multiple cerebral infarcts).
   2. Technique.
      a. IMP or HMPAO protocol.
      b. Quantitation (see below).
   3. Findings:
      a. Decreased uptake in the parietal lobes.
      b. Decreased uptake can be seen in the temporal, occipital, and frontal lobes as well.
      c. Cortical/cerebellar uptake ratio reduced from normal of 1 to <0.8.
        (1) Note: IMP may give erroneous ratios.
      d. Main differential is multiinfarct dementia, which shows multiple focal defects.
   4. Sensitivity and specificity.
      a. Quantitation improves sensitivity and specificity.
      b. Sensitivity overall—88%; specificity—87%.
        (1) Milder forms of the disease yielded a lower sensitivity—80%.
E. Psychiatric disorders.
   1. Much more work has been done with PET than with SPECT.
   2. A number of different patterns have been reported in schizophrenia.
F. Closed head injury.
   1. Background.
      a. Overall incidence approximately 200/100,000. This is similar to stroke and greater than epilepsy.
      b. Mortality from closed head injury is 34% to 49%, primarily in first 48 hours.
      c. Morbidity significant—neurologic loss.
      d. HMPAO can be helpful in detecting presence of morphologic abnormality.
   2. Technique.

      a. Routine HMPAO SPECT scan.

  3. Findings:

      a. Focal and/or diffuse decreased uptake.

  4. Sensitivity and specificity.

      a. Overall, sensitivity of HMPAO—80% vs. CT—55%.

      b. In patients with minor head injury, HMPAO sensitivity—60% vs. CT—25%.

G. Tumor.

  1. Determining grade of glioma.

      a. The degree of ^{201}Tl uptake in gliomas correlates with the histologic grade. Low uptake is seen with low-grade gliomas, higher uptake with high-grade gliomas.

  2. Differentiating glioma from postoperative changes and radiation necrosis.

      a. Tumor and radiation necrosis can appear similar on CT and MRI.

      b. Combination of ^{201}Tl and ^{99m}Tc HMPAO can be helpful in differentiating high-grade glioma from radiation necrosis.

      c. Technique.

        (1) Inject 3 mCI ^{201}Tl intravenously.

        (2) Perform SPECT.

        (3) Inject 20 mCi of ^{99m}Tc HMPAO.

        (4) Perform SPECT.

      d. Findings:

        (1) High ^{201}Tl and HMPAO uptake—tumor.

        (2) Moderate ^{201}Tl uptake and high HMPAO uptake—tumor.

        (3) Moderate ^{201}Tl uptake and decreased HMPAO uptake—radiation necrosis.

        (4) Low ^{201}Tl and HMPAO uptake—radiation necrosis.

CEREBROSPINAL FLUID IMAGING

Anatomy

(See beginning of Chapter 2.)

Physiology

(See beginning of Chapter 2.)

Radiopharmaceuticals

  I. ^{131}I Human serum albumin (RISA).

    A. Original material used for CSF studies.

    B. Cases of aseptic meningitis due to contamination with endotoxin.

II. DTPA
   A. Can be bound to indium 111 or technetium 99m.
   B. Most frequently used CSF agent.
   C. Infrequently associated with aseptic meningitis.
   D. Flows with CSF.
   E. Removed by arachnoid villi.
III. Ytterbium 169.
   A. Because of long half-life (32 days), delivers significantly higher radiation dose.
   B. Not recommended.

Technique

I. Injection.
   A. Lumbar puncture using 21- to 22-gauge spinal needle.
   B. 500 µCi of ^{111}In or mCi amounts of ^{99m}Tc injected.
   C. Can mix with 2 to 3 ml of 10% dextrose to make hyperbaric solution.
   D. Some also use Trendelenburg position.
   E. Fifteen percent of all injections extrathecal. Appears as wider, segmental appearance (normally a column); no activity is seen in basal cisterns at 3 hours. In these cases, must reinject.
II. Image 1, 4 to 6, 24, 48, and 72 hours. Anterior, posterior, laterals, vertex views. Parallel-hole medium-energy collimator set on 173/247 photopeaks. 50,000 to 100,000 count images. (^{99m}Tc set on 140-KeV photopeak.)

Normal Scan

I. Activity appears in basal cisterns by 3 hours, then enters interhemispheric and sylvian fissure forming Neptune's triumvirate.
II. Flow over convexities by 24 hours.
III. No reflux into ventricles is seen, although transient reflux at 12 to 24 hours not considered of significance.

Abnormal Scan

I. Hydrocephalus.
   A. Background.
      1. Increased CSF volume due to:
         a. Overproduction.
         b. Decreased absorption.
         c. Blockage of flow.
         d. Cerebral atrophy.
   B. Types.
      1. Nonobstructive.
         a. Due to cerebral atrophy.

2. Obstructive.
   a. Due to obstruction of outflow.
      (1) Noncommunicating hydrocephalus.
         (a) Due to internal blockage of egress of CSF.
      (2) Communicating obstructive hydrocephalus.
         (a) Due to extraventricular blockage (e.g., cisterns, villi).
C. Findings.
   1. Communicating hydrocephalus.
      a. Reflux into ventricles is primary finding. Capillaries in periventricular white matter become primary sites of absorption rather than arachnoid villae.
      b. Delayed flow over the convexities.
   2. Noncommunicating hydrocephalus.
      a. No ventricular reflux.
      b. Convexity flow—slow flow or normal.
II. Normal-pressure hydrocephalus (NPH).
   A. Background.
      1. Hydrocephalus with normal CSF pressures.
      2. Etiology unknown.
      3. Appears to start as a block to CSF flow/absorption.
      4. Symptoms:
         a. Triad of:
            (1) Dementia.
            (2) Gait disorder.
            (3) Urinary incontinence.
   B. Sensitivity.
      1. Relationship between CSF pattern and response to shunting is variable.
   C. Findings—variable.
      1. Ventricles—reflux that persists on 24-, 48-, and sometimes 72-hour views.
      2. Convexities—significantly delayed or lack of flow.
      3. Other patterns are abnormal but "indeterminate" for NPH.
III. Shunt patency.
   A. Background.
      1. CSF shunting system malfunctions are not uncommon.
      2. Disconnection of tubing, infection, and perforation of neighboring organs can occur. Ventriculoatrial shunts can cause superior venacaval thrombosis. Ventriculoperitoneal shunts can cause obstructions because of adhesions.
      3. ^{99m}Tc DTPA used.
      4. Instill in or near shunt and image.

      5. Activity reaching the vascular system or peritoneal cavity indicates free flow.

POSITRON EMISSION TOMOGRAPHY

I. Background.
    A. Two 511-keV photons emitted at 180° to each other on annihilation of a positron. Uses electronic collimation. Allows use of isotopes of carbon, nitrogen, and oxygen, the main constituents of the body.
II. Radiopharmaceuticals.
    A. Fluorine-18 fluorodeoxyglucose (FDG).
        1. A marker of glucose metabolism.
        2. Cyclotron-produced.
        3. Physical half-life—110 minutes.
        4. FDG is transported into cell by same carrier as glucose. Once inside the cell, it is phosphorylated by hexokinase. Further metabolism of DG-6-phosphate is blocked, and unlike glucose, does not proceed further in glycolytic pathway.
        5. The rate of glucose consumption per gram of tissue can be calculated.
    B. Nitrogen-13 ammonia.
        1. Regional cerebral blood flow marker.
        2. Cyclotron-produced.
        3. Circulates in blood as $^{13}NH_4^+$.
        4. Rapidly cleared from blood by myocardium and brain. Less than 2% remains in blood after administration.
        5. Efficiently extracted from the blood by the brain. Clears slowly—$T_{1/2}$ of 65 minutes.
        6. Cerebellar-to-subcortical white matter ratio—3.3.
    C. Oxygen-15 water.
        1. A marker of regional cerebral blood flow.
        2. Cyclotron-produced.
        3. Physical half-life—2 minutes.
        4. Freely diffuses across the cell membrane. Retention in cell is short, however, because agent rapidly equilibrates between tissue and vascular space.
    D. Carbon-11 and Fluorine-18 N-methylspiperone.
        1. A marker of neuroreceptor concentration.
        2. Cyclotron-produced.
        3. Binds to D2 dopamine receptors.
    E. Fluorine-18 fluoro-L-DOPA.
        1. A marker of neuroreceptors.
    F. Many more agents have been synthesized and are used for variety of purposes.

III. Uses.
  A. Many uses are similar to those discussed for SPECT agents.
  B. Cerebrovascular disease.
    1. PET is better able to track physiological events of stroke than other imaging techniques, including SPECT.
    2. Using nitrogen-13 ammonia and oxygen-15 labeled agents, the regional cerebral blood flow and oxygen metabolism have been studied.
      a. Early, decreased flow but increased oxygen extraction fraction occurs in an attempt to deliver maximal amount of oxygen to compromised region of brain.
      b. As stroke evolves, luxury perfusion stage develops. Flow increases in relation to oxygen extraction fraction.
      c. Additional hypometabolic foci distant from the infarction are often seen in absence of CT or MRI abnormalities. These abnormalities can be in the ipsilateral or contralateral hemisphere or in the contralateral cerebellar hemisphere. They are due to interruption of crossing pathways.
  C. Epilepsy.
    1. Findings similar to SPECT but more sensitive interictally than SPECT.
  D. Movement disorders.
    1. Huntington's disease.
      a. Decreased metabolism in caudate nucleii.
      b. Decreased D2 receptor density.
    2. Parkinson's disease.
      a. Reduced basal ganglia uptake of ^{18}F DOPA.
  E. Psychiatric disorders.
    1. Schizophrenia.
      a. Although many studies have shown decreased perfusion and metabolism of frontal lobes, some have not. Discrepancies in the age, chronicity of disease, subtype of schizophrenia, medications, and clinical state of patient at time of imaging may account for differences in findings among studies.
      b. Some studies have shown left hemisphere increased perfusion and metabolism.
      c. Some studies have shown an increased subcortical-to-cortical ratio.
    2. Mood disorders.
      a. Variable findings.
      b. Some evidence that depressed patients have globally diminished cerebral blood flow and metabolism.

      c. Some evidence for differences in scan appearance between unipolar and bipolar depressed patients.

F. Dementia.

    1. Findings similar to SPECT in Alzheimer's disease.

G. Brain tumors.

    1. As with SPECT, can determine grade of glioma and differentiate tumor from radiation necrosis.

    2. May see abnormalities away from tumor. Mechanism is similar to that discussed with stroke.

SUGGESTED READINGS

Alavi A, Hirsch LJ: Studies of central nervous system disorders with single-photon emission computed tomography and positron emission tomography: Evolution over the past two decades. *Semin Nucl Med* 1991; 21:58-81.

Bonte FJ, Hom J, Tintner R, et al: Single-photon tomography in Alzheimer's disease and the dementias. *Semin Nucl Med* 1990; 20:342-352.

Burt RW, Witt RM, Cikrit DF, et al: Carotid artery disease: Evaluation with acetazolamide-enhanced ^{99m}Tc HMPAO SPECT. *Radiol* 1992; 182:461-466.

Devous MD, Leroy RF, Homan RW: Single-photon emission computed tomography in epilepsy. *Semin Nucl Med* 1990; 20:325-341.

Falls M, Park CH, Madsen M: Iofetamine HCL I-123 (iodoamphetamine) brain SPECT atlas. *Clin Nucl Med* 1985; 10:443-449.

Gilday DL, Kellam J: ^{111}In-DTPA evaluation of CSF diversionary shunts in children. *J Nucl Med* 1973; 14:920-923. 1973.

Goodman JM, Heck LL, Moore BD, et al: Confirmation of brain death with portable isotope angiography: A review of 204 consecutive cases. *Neurosurgery* 1985; 16:492-497.

Graham P, Howman-Giles R, Johnston I, et al: Evaluation of CSF shunt patency by means of technetium-99m DTPA. *J Neurosurg* 1982; 56:262-266.

Gray BG, Ichise M, Chung DG, et al: [99m]Tc HMPAO SPECT in evaluation of patients with remote history of traumatic brain injury: A comparison with x-ray computed tomography. *J Nucl Med* 1992; 33:52-58.

Harbert J: Radionuclide cisternography. In Harbert J, Goncalves da Rocha F (eds): *Textbook of nuclear medicine.* Philadelphia, Lea & Febiger, 1984, pp 111-126.

Harbert JC: Radionuclide cisternography. *Semin Nucl Med* 1971; 1:90-106.

Harbert J: The brain. In Harbert J, Goncalves da Rocha F (eds): *Textbook of nuclear medicine.* Philadelphia, Lea & Febiger, 1984, pp. 73-110.

Hawkins RA, Kuhl DE, Phelps ME: Positron emission tomography of the brain. In Gottschalk A, Hoffer PB, Potchen EJ (eds): *Diagnostic nuclear medicine,* vol 2, Baltimore, Williams & Wilkins, 1988.

Hellman RS, Tikofsky RS: An overview of the contribution of regional cerebral blood flow studies in cerebrovascular disease: Is there a role for single-photon emission computed tomography? *Semin Nucl Med* 1990; 20:303-324.

Hill TC, Holman BL, Lovett R, et al: Initial experience with SPECT (single-photon computerized tomography) of the brain using N-isopropyl I-123 p-iodoamphetamine: Concise communication. *J Nucl Med* 1982; 23:191-195.

Hill TC, Magistretti PL, Holman BL, et al: Assessment of regional cerebral blood flow (r CBF) in stroke using SPECT and N-isopropyl-(I-123)-p-iodoamphetamine (IMP). *Stroke* 1984; 15:42-45.

Holman BL: Concepts and clinical utility of the measurement of cerebral blood flow. *Semin Nucl Med* 1976; 6:233-251.

Holman BL, Hill TC, Polak JF, et al: Cerebral perfusion imaging with iodine 123-labeled amines. *Arch Neurol* 1984; 41:1060-1063.

Holmes RA, Hawkins RA, Phelps ME, et al: The central nervous system. In Freeman LM (ed): *Freeman and Johnson's clinical radionuclide imaging*. New York, Grune & Stratton, 1984, p 611.

Kuhl DE, Barrio JR, Huang SC, et al: Quantifying local cerebral blood flow by N-isopropyl-p-[^{123}I] iodoamphetamine (IMP) tomography. *J Nucl Med* 1982; 23:196-203.

Lee RGL, Hill TC, Holman BL, et al: Comparison of N-Isopropyl (I-123) p-iodoamphetamine brain scans using Anger camera scintigraphy and single-photon emission tomography. *Radiology* 1982; 145:789-793.

Lee RGL, Hill TC, Holman BL, et al: N-isopropyl (I-123) p-iodoamphetamine brain scans with single-photon emission tomography: Discordance with transmission computed tomography. *Radiology* 1982; 145:795-799.

McKusick KA, Malmud LS, Kordela PA, et al: Radionuclide cisternography: Normal values for nasal secretion of intrathecally-injected ^{111}In-DTPA. *J Nucl Med* 1973; 14:933-934.

Perani D, DiPiero V, Vallar G, et al: ^{99m}Tc HMPAO SPECT study of regional cerebral perfusion in early Alzheimer's disease. *J Nucl Med* 1988; 29:1507-1514.

Peterman SB, Taylor AT, Hoffman JC: Improved detection of cerebral hypoperfusion with internal carotid balloon test occlusion and ^{99m}Tc HMPAO cerebral perfusion SPECT imaging. *AJNR* 1991; 12:1035-1041.

Reivich M, Alavi A (eds): *Positron emission tomography,* New York, Alan R. Liss, 1985.

de la Riva A, Gonzalez FM, Llamas-Elvira JM, et al: Diagnosis of brain death: Superiority of perfusion studies with ^{99m}Tc HMPAO over conventional radionuclide cerebral angiography. *Brit J Radiol* 1992; 65:289-294.

Royal HD, Hill TC, Holman BL: Clinical brain imaging with isopropyl-iodoamphetamine and SPECT. *Semin Nucl Med* 1985; 25:357-376.

Schwartz RB, Carvalho PA, Alexander E, et al: Radiation necrosis vs high-grade recurrent glioma: Differentiation by using dual-isotope SPECT with ^{201}Tl and ^{99m}Tc HMPAO. *AJNR* 1992; 12:1187-1192.

3
Bone Imaging

BONE
Anatomy and Physiology

I. In mature bone, outer cortex of compact bone is present with inner surface of loose trabecular-cancellous bone. Architecture arranged in haversian system.

II. Bone surrounded by periosteal membrane except for articular surfaces. Periosteum contains capillaries that penetrate cortex to medullary canal. In children, periosteum more vascular and loosely attached to bone than in adults.

III. Three cell types in bone:
   A. Osteoblast—produce bone matrix—organic.
   B. Osteocyte—synthesize bone matrix—inorganic.
   C. Osteoclast—active in bone resorption.

IV. Two types of ossification.
   A. Endochondral—replacement of cartilaginous tissues by bone at ossification centers.
   B. Intramembranous ossification—mesenchymal cells differentiate into osteoblasts that deposit amorphous ground substance. Blasts trapped within lacunae become osteocytes and lay down a matrix.

V. Bone primarily composed of:
   A. Organic matrix.
      1. Collagen.
      2. Mucopolysaccharides.
   B. Inorganic matrix.
      1. Hydroxyapatite.
      2. Cations.
         a. Calcium.
         b. Magnesium.
         c. Sodium.
         d. Potassium.
         e. Strontium.
      3. Anions.
         a. Phosphorous.

b. Chlorine.

c. Fluorine.

VI. Osteogenesis and bone resorption continually occur even in normal bone.

Radiopharmaceuticals

I. Calcium 47.

A. Calcium major cation found in bone.

B. Unfortunately, radioisotopes of calcium have poor imaging characteristics. Calcium 47 decays by beta particle emission with release 1.3 MeV gamma photon.

C. High-energy photons.

1. Detected with poor counting efficiency.

2. Collimator septal penetration degrades spatial resolution.

II. Strontium 85 (^{85}Sr).

A. First radionuclide widely used for bone imaging.

B. Calcium analogue administered in ionic form and is taken up in bone by:

1. Diffusion into outer hydration shell in exchange with ionic calcium. Exchange reaction takes only minutes.

2. Exchange with ions at crystal surface.

3. Intracrystalline ion incorporation at sites of new bone formation.

C. 50% injected dose incorporated into bone within 1 hour. Remainder excreted by:

1. Kidneys.

2. Gastrointestinal (GI) tract—because of GI activity, imaging routinely performed 5 to 7 days after administration.

D. Disadvantages.

1. High radiation absorbed dose.

2. High energy gamma emission (514 keV) yielded poor imaging characteristics.

3. Delayed imaging time necessary.

III. Strontium 87 m (^{87m}Sr).

A. Produced by decay of yttrium 87 (^{87}Y) (80-hour half-life); decays by EC and positron emission.

B. Obtained by generator.

C. Lower-energy gamma ray—388 keV; shorter half-life—2.8 hours—improvement over ^{85}Sr.

D. Disadvantages

1. Because of short half-life, must be imaged 2 to 3 hours after injection. Low target-to-background ratios at this time due to slow blood and soft-tissue clearance.

IV. Fluorine 18.

A. Decays by positron emission—two 511-keV gamma photons produced by annihilation.
B. 50% of administered dose incorporated in calcium hydroxyapatite crystal via exchange with hydroxyl radicals, which are similar in physical size to fluorine.
C. Rapid renal excretion results in high bone-to-blood ratios 2 to 3 hours after administration.
D. Disadvantages.
   1. Short half-life makes delivery to institutions distant from site of production difficult.
   2. High cost.
   3. Imaging requires special equipment.
V. Technetium 99m phosphate compounds—most commonly used agents.
   A. Condensed phosphates.
      1. ^{99m}Tc triphosphate.
         a. First technetium phosphate bone agent introduced.
         b. Inorganic compound composed of three phosphate residues containing P-O-P bonds.
         c. High avidity for bone localization and good renal excretion of activity not localized in bone results in high target-to-background activity.
      2. ^{99m}Tc polyphosphate.
         a. Next agent to be introduced, superior to triphosphate.
         b. Long-chain phosphate residue up to 46 units.
      3. ^{99m}Tc pyrophosphate.
         a. Contains two phosphate residues.
         b. Superior in localization in infarcted tissues to other bone agents commonly used today.
   B. Diphosphonate.
      1. Organic analogues of pyrophosphate characterized by P-C-P bond.
      2. Numerous advantages over condensed phosphates including:
         a. Not susceptible to enzymatic hydrolysis in vivo by pyrophosphatases, etc.
         b. Lower percentage of plasma protein binding enhancing renal excretion.
            (1) ^{99m}Tc polyphosphate 68% to 84% protein bound at 3 hours after injection compared with 10% ^{99m}Tc methylene diphosphonate (see below).
         c. Have negligible red blood cell binding in distinction to pyrophosphates, which have 1% to 15% binding to red blood cells by 1 to 3 hours.
      3. Major diphosphonate agents.

    a. ^{99m}Tc HEDP—hydroxyethylene diphosphonate.

    b. ^{99m}Tc MDP—methylene diphosphonate.

        (1) At 1 hour, 58% of dose in bone.

        (2) At 6 hours, 68% compared with 48% HEDP; 47% pyrophosphate.

        (3) Cumulative 6-hour urinary excretion MDP, 68%; HEDP—68%; pyrophosphate—50%; polyphosphate, 46%.

    c. ^{99m}Tc HMDP—hydroxymethylene diphosphonate.

C. Imidodiphosphonates.

    1. Polyphosphate compounds containing P-N-P bonds.

    2. Not widely used at present for bone imaging.

D. Mechanisms of phosphate uptake in bone.

    1. Chemisorption.

        a. Absorption via chemical bonding.

        b. Occurs at kink and dislocation sites on surface of hydroxyapatite crystals. Tin and ^{99m}Tc released. These are hydrolyzed and bind to bone either separately or together as hydrated tin oxide and technetium dioxide.

        c. Large surface areas, such as growth center and reactive bone lesions, allow enhanced chemisorption.

    2. Organic matrix.

        a. Less commonly held theory is phosphate complexes bind primarily to immature collagen rather than bone crystals.

    3. Enzyme and enzyme receptor sites.

        a. Small contribution to binding.

        b. Occurs in organic matrix of bone.

        c. Alkaline phosphatase, etc.

E. Physiologic determinants of uptake of phosphate agents.

    1. Metabolic activity.

        a. Bony turnover most important determinant of uptake of radiopharmaceuticals.

        b. Related in large part to blood flow, as well as large surface area.

        c. Accounts for increased uptake seen at growth centers, osteoblastic lesions, etc.

    2. Blood flow.

        a. Flow must be present for delivery of radiopharmaceutical. If not, produces cold bone defects.

        b. With increased blood flow, increased deposition, although not linear at high rates. With three to four times increased flow, deposition increases 30% to 40%. This is diffusion-limited response.

3. Sympathetic tone.
  a. Responsible for closing capillaries.
  b. Following sympathectomy, vessels opened resulting in local increased blood flow—recruitment.
  c. This results in increased tracer accumulation following stroke or hemiplegia.
  d. Osteomyelitis, fractures, and tumor may also impair interosseous sympathetics, resulting in a hyperemic effect. Less important, however, than increased bone turnover rate.
F. Preparation of phosphate bone agents.
  1. Technetium 99m eluted from molybdenum 99 generator in Tc(7+) oxidation state as pertechnetate ion (^{99m}Tc O$_4^-$). If mixed with phosphate agents, no binding occurs. For binding, technetium must be reduced.
  2. Stannous chloride (Sn[II]) is used to chemically reduce technetium-pertechnetate to TC(4+) oxidation state. This causes a ^{99m}Tc-Sn phosphate complex to form that will localize in bone.
  3. Important that oxygen not be introduced into mixing vial during preparation of phosphate radiopharmaceuticals, since oxidation of technetium will result in poor tagging.
  4. Bone radiopharmaceuticals should be checked by chromatography before use. 90% to 95% + tagging necessary.
  5. Tag will break down with time; therefore, kits should not be used after approximately 4 hours after preparation time.

Technique

I. Patient is encouraged to maintain good hydration prior to scanning.
II. Four-phase bone scan.
  A. Performed when infection present. With tumor, often only static images or combination of first three phases obtained.
  B. Flow study.
    1. Patient is given 20 mCi of ^{99m}Tc MDP injected IV. Sequential images are obtained every 3 seconds for 60 seconds. These are imaged over the area of clinical concern.
  C. Blood pool.
    1. Immediately following the flow study, a blood pool image is obtained over the area of interest for 500,000 counts.
  D. Static images.
    1. After a minimum of 2 hours' delay (longer delays improve target-to-background ratio), multiple images are obtained over the skeleton. Large-field-of-view camera using a parallel-hole high-resolution collimator is used. Initial anterior view over the thorax for 400,000 counts is obtained. The time for this scan is recorded and all subsequent images are done for this

time. If the fourth phase is to be obtained, a 100,000 count over the area of interest is obtained.
E. 24-hour view.
1. A delayed image at 24 hours is obtained over the area of concern; 100,000 counts are recorded.
III. Sacral lesions.
A. Tail on detector (TOD) view for evaluating sacral lesions is used when bladder activity is superimposed over the sacrum (or pubis) on routine views. Usually obtained not by having patients sit on camera (which can crack the crystal), but by having patients get on hands and knees or scan through Lucite table.
IV. Whole body imaging.
A. Use dual-headed camera with high resolution, low energy parallel-hole collimators.
B. Set matrix for 256 × 1024.
C. Scan for 30 minutes using both heads.
V. SPECT imaging.
A. Settings vary with number of heads.
B. Dual-headed camera—high resolution, low energy parallel-hole collimators.
C. 128 × 128 matrix; magnification—1.00.
D. 360 degree (180 degree per head) acquisition using 60 steps/head; 30 seconds/stop.
VI. Pediatric patients.
A. Minimum dose—2 mCi (250 µCi/kg).
B. Pinhole views are often required, *especially* in cases of suspected osteomyelitis.

Normal Scan

I. Symmetry is sine qua non of normal bone scan.
II. Areas with normally increased activity on bone scan include:
A. Acromioclavicular joints.
B. Sternoclavicular joints.
C. Scapular tips.
D. Costochondral junctions.
E. Sacroiliac joints.
F. Normal lordosis of cervical lumbar spine causes increased activity in lower neck on anterior views.
G. Sternum has variable appearance.
H. Uptake in frontal and parasagittal areas commonly seen.
III. Adults
A. The bones are well seen with minimal soft-tissue activity.
B. Both kidneys are seen with mild activity. Renal pelves or

calyces are sometimes identified. Urinary bladder is almost always seen.

  1. *If* imaging has been delayed for 4 hours or more, the kidneys may not be seen. In addition, soft-tissue activity will be virtually absent, leading to the false diagnosis of "beautiful bone scan, or superscan."

C. Normal variants.

  1. Deltoid tuberosity—7% of patients show uptake in proximal humerus where deltoid muscle inserts. May be asymmetrical.
  2. Linear activity running along ribs posteriorly in a vertical orientation due to insertion of the iliocostalis thoracis portion of the erector spinae muscle group—prominent in 7%.
  3. Lower part of neck—may be caused by normal cervical lordosis or uptake in thyroid cartilage.

D. Pitfalls.

  1. Patient rotation—often makes iliac wings, and less commonly other areas, appear asymmetric and thus abnormal.
  2. Urine retained in calyx may overlie lower rib, simulating a bony lesion. Upright, oblique, and delayed viewed will show activity is renal.
  3. Patients, especially males, frequently contaminate clothing with radioactive urine. Activity usually overlies soft tissues but may overlie bony structures. Views with clothing removed and obliqued will show activity is on skin. Can also wash off skin, although if activity has been present for some time, often cannot be removed.
  4. Belt buckles, earrings, necklaces, and the like frequently create cold defects.
  5. Breast prostheses will give asymmetrical activity over chest.
  6. Recent dental procedures and dental disease frequently cause uptake in mandible and maxilla.
  7. Degenerative disease frequently causes uptake in joints.
  8. Radiopharmaceutical problems.
      a. Breakdown of tag leading to free pertechnetate causes activity to be seen in thyroid and GI tract.
      b. If colloid is formed, reticuloendothelial (RES) system seen.
      c. Material may be excreted in biliary system.

IV. Pediatric patients.

A. Increased uptake in growth centers. On normal bone scan, margins of growth plate clearly demarcated. Any irregularity or asymmetry should be viewed with suspicion. Especially important since osteomyelitis and neuroblastoma metastases have predilection for this region.

B. Ischiopubic synchondrosis—fixed joint between distal ends of inferior pubic and ischial ramae. Mass of cartilage that ossifies between ages 4 and 12. If fusion asymmetric and nonfused site still shows uptake, may be confused with abnormal uptake.

C. Increased uptake in cranial sutures normally seen.

Abnormal Scans

I. Increased uptake in areas outside of those normally known to show increased tracer accumulation.

II. Areas of decreased activity.

III. Disease processes.

A. Metastatic disease.

  1. Tumors most likely to metastasize to bone include:

    a. Breast.

    b. Lung.

    c. Prostate.

    d. Lymphoma.

    e. Thyroid.

    f. Renal.

    g. Neuroblastoma.

  2. Bone scanning significantly more sensitive than plain radiographs for detection of metastases. Negative radiographic findings found in 30% to 50% of patients with positive bone scan. This related to fact that approximately 30% to 50% of bone mineral must be lost before a lesion can be detected by conventional radiography.

    a. Note that approximately 5% of patients with negative bone scans will have positive radiographs. This related to low metabolic activity in lesion. Tumors in which falsely normal bone scan can be expected include:

      (1) Multiple myeloma.

      (2) Thyroid cancer.

      (3) Some anaplastic tumors.

      (4) Pure lytic lesions.

  3. Alkaline and acid phosphatase and serum calcium levels relatively insensitive as early indicators for presence of metastatic disease. Example: in prostate carcinoma, if bone scan sensitivity = 1, alkaline phosphatase sensitivity = 0.54 to 0.77; serum acid phosphatase = 0.5 to 0.6.

  4. Pain often late manifestation of metastatic disease. In one series of patients with prostatic carcinoma, 45% reported no pain at time of discovery of metastases. Complicating the issue, 12% of those without bony metastases complained of bone pain.

5. Approximately 90% of metastases are multiple.
6. Location of metastases:
   a. Axial skeleton—80%.
      (1) Vertebrae—39%.
      (2) Ribs and sternum—28%.
      (3) Pelvis—12%.
   b. Skull—10%.
   c. Long bones—10%. More commonly situated in proximal rather than distal portion of long bones.
7. Solitary lesions.
   a. Overall, 50% solitary lesions in patients with known tumor are malignant. Location helpful.
   b. Rib—malignant in 10% to 17% (Note this is in patients with known extraskeletal malignancy). The rest are:
      (1) 40% benign traumatic fractures.
      (2) 27% radiation therapy.
      (3) 24% unknown.
   d. Skull—20% due to metastatic disease.
      (1) Majority benign lesions in skull found in regions of sutures—postulated because of small cartilaginous rests.
8. Super scan or beautiful bone scan.
   a. Bone scan in which diffuse symmetrical increased uptake occurs. Clues that alert one to super scan include:
      (1) Almost total absence of soft-tissue activity.
      (2) Lack of kidney activity.
      (3) Uptake seen on early blood pool images.
   b. Tumors frequently causing super scan:
      (1) Prostate—most common.
      (2) Breast.
      (3) Lung.
      (4) Bladder.
      (5) Lymphoma.
   c. Nontumor causes of super scan.
      (1) Hyperparathyroidism.
      (2) Osteomalacia.
      (3) Paget's disease.
      (4) Fibrous dysplasia.
   d. Can differentiate cause of superscan, metabolic disease versus metastases, by the involvement of calvarium and long bones in metabolic bone disease in distinction to metastases, which tend to spare them.
9. False-positive scans.
   a. Although sensitive, bone scans are nonspecific. Any cause

of increased metabolic activity, whether resulting from metastatic disease, primary bone tumor, inflammatory disease, or trauma, can cause increased uptake.

b. Most common problem is degenerative joint disease (DJD). Location near a joint and degree of uptake is helpful indicator. Plain films will confirm. In one study 11% of patients had metastases in regions of DJD, however.

c. Next most common cause is trauma. Old fractures can remain hot for years.

   (1) Compression fractures—usually show a linear band of activity. Cannot differentiate with certainty from metastasis causing collapse.

   (2) Rib fractures.

      (a) Linear activity involving several ribs is almost certain indicator of trauma.

      (b) Discrete circular activity more likely to be fracture than long linear activity.

      (c) Activity near anterior rib tips almost always traumatic.

      (d) Plain films helpful if they show fracture. Lack of fracture on film does not completely rule out trauma, however, especially near costochondral junctions.

10. Following treatment response.

a. Signs of progression include an increase in number, extent, or degree of activity in bone lesions. Improvement shown by opposite changes.

b. Stable scans, showing no change, are not necessarily a sign of unfavorable response. Shown to have improved survival similar to patients whose scans show improvement.

c. Flare phenomenon.

   (1) Lesions increase in activity on scan (similar to osteoblastic response seen on plain films) in response to treatment. This is thought to be due to:

      (a) Increased blood flow caused by inflammatory response.

      (b) Increased turnover of hydroxyapatite in new bone laid down as part of healing.

   (2) Fortunately, appears to be uncommon.

   (3) Follow-up scan 3 months later can be helpful if not certain.

B. Primary malignant bone tumors.

1. Osteogenic sarcoma.

a. Usually occurs in second decade.

b. Half located in region of knee.

    c. Other sites include:
      (1) Long bone metaphyses.
      (2) Skull.
      (3) Mandible.
      (4) Ileum.
      (5) Spine.
      (6) Scapula.
    d. Approximately 25% at autopsy have skeletal metastases.
    e. Bone scan demonstrates increased vascularity on flow and delayed uptake that is very intense.
  2. Chondrosarcoma.
    a. Half of patients older than 40. Rare in children.
    b. Characteristically present with joint pain.
    c. Tumors located in epiphyseal ossification center of long bones.
    d. Increased blood flow, blood pool, and uptake on delayed images seen at tumor site. Uptake related to increased blood flow and tumoral calcifications in peripheral chondrosarcomas.
  3. Ewing's sarcoma.
    a. Peak incidence first to second decades.
    b. Arises from bone marrow elements.
    c. Clinical manifestations similar to osteomyelitis—pain, fever, leukocytosis.
    d. Femur and tibia, and other long bones of extremities, primary sites.
    e. At autopsy 60% have bone metastases.
    f. Increased uptake on delayed images usual finding.
C. Benign primary tumors.
  1. Osteoid osteoma.
    a. Age—second to third decades.
    b. Clinical—aching pain, worse at night, relieved with aspirin and exercise.
    c. Location—cortically based in tubular bones. Spine common site. When involved, usually posterior elements rather than vertebral body. Can cause painful scoliosis with the apex at lesion, concave on side of lesion.
    d. Scan sensitivity—excellent. Negative scan virtually rules out osteoid osteoma.
    e. Findings.
      (1) Blood pool-increased activity almost invariably.
      (2) Delayed—focal, usually intense, increased uptake.
      (3) May have double-density sign—focally hotter area surrounded by less intense but increased activity. Focal

hotter area represents nidus. May be centrally or eccentrically located.

2. Bone islands.
   a. Usually normal or minimal uptake.
   b. Detection depends on:
      (1) Size—≥3 cm.
      (2) Growth rate.
      (3) Lesion location.

3. Bone cysts.
   a. Normal or minimal activity.
   b. More intense uptake usually indicates fracture through cyst.

4. Fibrous cortical defects, nonossifying fibroma.
   a. Normal or minimal uptake.
   b. Blood flow studies negative.

5. Other benign lesions.
   a. Multiple other benign lesions can show increased uptake. Total body imaging is helpful for diagnosed multiplicity.
      (1) Fibrous dysplasia.
      (2) Eosinophilic granuloma.
      (3) Brown tumors of hyperparathyroidism.
      (4) Aneurysmal bone cysts.
      (5) Chondroblastoma.
      (6) Enchondroma.

D. Osteomyelitis.
   1. Background.
      a. Acute hematogenous osteomyelitis usually occurs in children. Less common in adults. Approximately one-half have history of superficial staphylococcal infection.
      b. Usually located in diaphyseal/epiphyseal region. In children, growing end of the epiphyses represents greatest blood flow to bone. Also, end-arterial circulation of diaphysis is important. Spread into adjacent joints is uncommon, except in infants in whom growth plate does not serve as effective barrier.
      c. Infection spreads along periosteum or marrow cavity. Eventually penetrates cortex through haversian system. Increased pressure, or stripping of periosteum by pus, may produce local ischemia (cold defect).
      d. Most common sites include:
         (1) About knee (distal femur, proximal tibia).
         (2) About ankle (distal tibia, distal fibula).
         (3) Humerus, head and distal portion.
         (4) Calcaneous.

    e. Blood cultures positive in 50% of cases.

    f. Plain films usually normal for first 10 to 14 days.

    g. Bone scan sensitivity—76% to 91%. Similar specificities. Note that sensitivity may be decreased at extremes of age (neonates less than 6 months and elderly patients). In addition, concomitant antibiotic therapy may decrease sensitivity as well. Note scan usually positive within first 24 hours of symptoms.

2. Findings.

    a. Osteomyelitis.

        (1) Flow—increased.

        (2) Blood pool—increased.

        (3) Delayed—increased. Note that bone/soft tissue ratio in lesion increases with time up to 24 hours. Uptake usually more focal than in cellulitis.

    b. Cellulitis.

        (1) Flow—increased; especially localized to soft tissues.

        (2) Blood pool—increased.

        (3) Delayed—usually shows mild diffuse increased activity. May show *mild* focal activity. With delayed imaging, bone/soft tissue ratio falls.

    c. Cold bone defects.

        (1) Seen in early osteomyelitis because of:

            (a) Increased pressure reducing blood flow.

            (b) Stripping away of periosteum via pus.

            (c) Interruption of blood supply via sludging and thrombosis.

        (2) Increased danger of sequestrum formation.

        (3) Will usually become transformed into hot lesion. In process, may go through stage of normal degree of activity.

        (4) Especially difficult to diagnose in flat bones.

3. Other radiopharmaceuticals for osteomyelitis.

    a. Gallium 67.

        (1) Acute osteomyelitis.

            (a) Thought to be more sensitive for osteomyelitis than bone scan; therefore, if bone scan negative and high clinical suspicion, gallium scan should follow.

            (b) Findings—increased uptake in region of bone.

            (c) Fractures, recent bone surgery, etc., also show uptake.

            (d) Gallium may show incongruence with bone scan in patients with recent fracture or orthopedic procedure if osteomyelitis present, i.e., gallium uptake in region of bone not showing increased uptake on bone scan or more intense uptake in an area than is seen on bone scan. This indicates osteomyelitis. Unfortunately, majority of patients, even with osteomyelitis, will show congruence between scans.

(2) Chronic osteomyelitis.

    (a) Useful when compared with bone scan, to diagnose reactivation chronic osteomyelitis. Will see gallium incongruence. Note congruence does not definitely rule out osteomyelitis, but makes it less likely.

(3) Osteomyelitis versus cellulitis.

    (a) Gallium will localize more in soft tissues, since not dependent on blood flow as much as polymorphonuclear infiltration, etc. May be helpful, therefore, in differentiating cellulitis from osteomyelitis.

(4) Septic arthritis.

    (a) Gallium uptake localized to soft tissue of joint more than bones themselves in septic arthritis. Helpful in differentiating osteomyelitis from septic arthritis.

(5) Gallium response to therapy.

    (a) Bone scan remains hot due to healing phase even in treated osteomyelitis. Gallium tends to fade with successful therapy; however, utility not definitely established.

    (b) Radiolabeled leukocytes.

        (i) Many centers use labeled leukocytes rather than ^{67}Ga for osteomyelitis.

           a Gallium 67 is a weak bone agent; this makes interpretation difficult in patients of postorthopedic surgery. Labeled leukocytes do not normally accumulate in these sites.

        (ii) Evidence exists that labeled leukocytes are less sensitive for vertebral osteomyelitis than for other sites of osteomyelitis.

E. Septic arthritis.

  1. Findings.

    a. Flow increased in soft tissue of joint.

    b. Increased in blood pool around joint. Note: Does not extend greatly into bone.

    c. Increased uptake diffusely in bones around joint.

F. Diabetic osteoarthropathy and foot ulcers.

1. Findings.
   a. Flow—increased.
   b. Blood pool—increased.
   c. Delayed—increased activity in bone near ulcer and joints affected by diabetic osteoarthropathy. Usually bone/soft tissue ratio falls with time although may not.
G. Prosthetic joints.
   1. Complications causing pain include:
      a. Loosening.
      b. Infection.
      c. Heterotopic bone formation.
      d. Inflammatory bursitis.
      e. Breakage of fixation wires.
      f. Fracture/dislocation prosthesis.
   2. Scan especially helpful in differentiating loosening from infection. However, should start with plain films since, if abnormal, can stop. Because scan more sensitive, should be next step.
   3. Normal scan.
      a. No evidence of increased flow or blood pool.
      b. Photopenic area corresponding to prosthesis.
      c. Delayed—often see increased uptake around prosthesis for 9 to 12 months. Some uptake up to 36 months has been reported in occasional patients.
      d. Increased activity in region of greater or lesser trochanter should be considered normal.
      e. Can use opposite hip as control if it does not have a prosthesis.
   4. Findings.
      a. Loosening.
         (1) Blood flow and blood pools—normal.
         (2) Delayed images—increased uptake around prosthesis—usually focal at tip of femoral component. Diffuse uptake *may* be seen but more likely to be seen in infection. Remember that infection causes loosening.
      b. Infection.
         (1) Blood flow and blood pool—increased.
         (2) Delayed images—increased uptake more diffusely around prosthesis than usually seen with loosening.
      c. Heterotopic bone formation.
         (1) Increased uptake on delayed images outside of bone. Often parallels prosthetic femoral neck.
      d. Bursitis.
         (1) Increased flow, blood pool, and statics outside of normal confines of bone.

5. Labeled leukocytes are also useful for diagnosing infection. They have a high sensitivity and specificity in prosthetic patients.

a. Occasionally bone marrow is pushed down by a femoral prosthesis and will cause a focal area of leukocyte uptake at the tip of the prosthesis. A bone marrow scan using ^{99m}Tc sulfur colloid can differentiate compressed marrow from infection.

H. Fracture.

1. Traumatic fracture.

a. Will become positive within 24 hours because of repair processes.

(1) 80% abnormal by 24 hours.

(2) 95% abnormal by 72 hours.

(3) 98% abnormal by 1 week. Note that it takes longer for the scans of older patients to become abnormal.

b. Resolution time.

(1) Approximately two-thirds return to normal by 1 year—minimum 5 to 7 months.

(2) 90% normal by 2 years.

(a) Approximately 10% remain abnormal for 3 or more years. Especially seen in fractures of long bone with callous formation and repeated bone stress.

(3) Scan can be used to pick up old fractures such as in spine, etc.

(4) May also be used in child abuse to detect fractures. Problems:

(a) Will not detect old, healed fractures.

(b) Difficult to evaluate around metaphyseal/epiphyseal region.

(c) May miss some skull fractures.

2. Stress fractures.

a. Two types.

(1) Fatigue fractures—caused by repeated abnormal stress on normal bone, such as with runners.

(a) Much more sensitive than plain film.

(b) Findings.

(i) If acute (less than 1 month) increased flow and blood pool.

(ii) Increased uptake on delayed images. Pattern is:

a Fusiform, longitudinal shape, most often involving posterior tibial cortex.

Helpful if it extends more than half through width of bone.

b Focal, runs less than one-fifth length of tibia.

c Common location is junction of middle and distal third of tibia.

(c) Stress fracture usually must be differentiated from shin splints. Shin splints thought to be related to abnormal stress of soleus muscle at tibial origin. Findings of shin splints are:

(i) Radionuclide angiogram and blood pools—normal.

(ii) Delayed—linear, longitudinal area of activity confined to posterior tibial cortex.

(iii) Longer length of bone involved, one third to three fourths.

(iv) Commonly located distal portion middle third of tibia to proximal portion of distal third of tibia.

(2) Insufficiency fractures—resulting from normal stress on abnormal bone.

(a) Seen in such diseases as:

(i) Osteoporosis.

(ii) Osteomalacia.

(iii) Paget's disease.

(iv) Fibrous dysplasia.

(v) Status postirradiation.

(b) Often difficult to diagnose on plain films because of underlying bone disease.

(c) Bone scan especially helpful for sacral insufficiency fractures. Appear as bilateral linear areas of increased uptake in region of sacral alae.

I. Metabolic bone disease.

1. Osteoporosis.

a. Most common metabolic bone disease.

b. Scan frequently normal.

c. With severe osteoporsis, may see decreased uptake.

d. Disuse osteoporosis.

(1) Frequently associated with positive scans (diffuse increased uptake).

(2) In first several years of disuse, bone formation increases twice normal, although resorption increases even more.

    e. Regional migratory osteoporosis.

        (1) Middle-aged men.

        (2) Present with joint pain, especially hip.

        (3) Findings.

            (a) Increased blood flow on angiogram.

            (b) Increased periarticular uptake in involved joint, which may migrate to other joints on serial scans.

2. Osteomalacia.

    a. Due to vitamin D deficiency. Results in failure of bone matrix to calcify

    b. Bone scan findings—generalized increased skeletal uptake common finding.

3. Hyperparathyroidism.

    a. Primary hyperparathyroidism.

        (1) Caused by hyperplasia or tumor of parathyroids (adenoma or rarely carcinoma) causing excessive secretion of parathyroid hormone.

        (2) Biochemically—increased serum calcium, decreased serum phosphate, increased serum alkaline phosphatase, increased serum parathyroid hormone.

        (3) Findings.

            (a) 50% to 80% of patients have normal bone scan appearance.

            (b) Those abnormal show:

                (i) Uptake at areas that radiographically show demineralization or erosion. These include:

                    a Calvarium (particularly periphery).

                    b Mandible.

                    c Acromioclavicular joint.

                    d Sternum.

                    e Lateral humeral epicondyles

                    f Hands.

                (ii) Brown tumors, if present, may accumulate bone agent.

                (iii) Soft-tissue calcification shows uptake in:

                    a Lungs.

                    b Stomach.

                    c Kidneys.

                    d Heart.

                    e Periarticular.

    b. Secondary hyperparathyroidism.

        (1) Usually associated with chronic renal failure. Excessive

destruction of renal parenchyma occurs, preventing 25-hydroxy-cholecalciferol from being hydroxylated to its 1,25-hydroxy form. This results in vitamin D deficiency. In addition, rise in phosphate with decreased glomerular filtration rate (GFR) causes feedback, increasing parathormone secretion.

    (2) Unlike primary, secondary usually does have abnormal bone scan.

    (3) Findings.

        (a) Super scan.

        (b) Focal abnormalities seen in same areas as with primary. In addition, may show increased activity of proximal and distal phalanges and metacarpals, as well as costochondral regions similar to childhood rickets.

4. Paget's disease.

  a. One of the most common chronic skeletal diseases—affects 3% of people older than 40 years of age.

  b. Cause—unknown. May be viral etiology.

  c. Pathophysiology—increased resorption of bone accompanied by increase in bone formation. However, newly formed bone is abnormally soft and exhibits disorganized trabecular pattern with larger number of cellular and vascular spaces.

  d. Skeletal pain most frequent symptom; however, many patients asymptomatic.

  e. Complications include:

    (1) Pathologic fracture.

    (2) Degenerative joint disease.

    (3) Malignant transformation—osteosarcoma (occurs in less than 1% of patients).

  f. Radiographically, lesions of Paget's begin as lytic lesion. With maturation, become blastic. Ultimately, sclerotic pattern often appears. At this point, disease may have become quiescent and osteoblastic activity ceases.

  g. Sensitivity—60% of lesions seen both scintigraphically and radiographically; 27% seen only on scan; 13% seen only on radiographs.

  h. Bone scan shows increased uptake, largely due to significant increase in blood flow associated in Paget's bone.

  i. Findings.

    (1) Increased uptake in bones usually involved by Paget's (see above).

       (2) Activity involves entire bone or large portion of bone.

       (3) In osteoporosis circumscripta phase, may see colder center with increased activity at the edge of lesion.

       (4) May be negative in sclerotic phase due to lack of osteoblastic activity.

   j. Distribution of lesions.

       (1) Pelvis most frequently involved, 70% to 80%.

       (2) Lumbar-thoracic vertebrae.

       (3) Femur.

       (4) Skull.

       (5) Scapula.

       (6) Tibia.

       (7) Humerus.

   k. Especially important to think of Paget's in scans for metastases, because it occurs so frequently and may be asymptomatic.

J. Avascular necrosis.

  1. Adults.

    a. Avascular necrosis may occur as a result of:

       (1) Fracture.

       (2) Metabolic disorder.

       (3) Fat embolization.

       (4) Steroids.

       (5) Hemolytic anemias.

       (6) Vasculitis.

    b. Early, plain film is normal. Radiographic changes of avascular necrosis after subcapital fracture of femoral neck may not be evident for 6 months.

    c. Immediately following fracture, bone scans may be normal for first 48 hours, then show decreased activity for variable period followed by increasing activity as reparative processes occur. In addition, patients may develop degenerative joint disease due to avascular necrosis and show increased uptake in the acetabulum simulating uptake in the femoral head. Therefore, radionuclide diagnosis of avascular necrosis with bone scan may be difficult.

    d. SPECT has higher sensitivity for AVN than planar images.

       (1) Comparison of planar and SPECT imaging found that planar had a sensitivity of 55%, compared to 85% for SPECT imaging.

       (2) A cold central defect is seen with surrounding increased activity.

       (3) If a central cold focus is not identified because of

increased uptake in surrounding humoral head and acetabulum, AVN cannot be differentiated from osteoarthritis, inflammatory arthritis, fracture, or other osseous abnormalities.

K. Legg-Calvé-Perthes disease.
  1. Primarily affects boys aged 4 to 8 years.
  2. Necrosis of femoral capital epiphyses occurs, likely due to vascular origin.
  3. Sensitivity—98%; specificity—95%.
  4. Findings.
      a. Decreased activity in femoral capital epiphysis.
      b. Increased activity in acetabulum (caused by associated synovitis).
      c. Increased activity found if subsequent revascularization and healing has occurred.

L. Reflex sympathetic dystrophy syndrome.
  1. Syndrome consists of:
      a. Pain.
      b. Tenderness.
      c. Vasomotor instability.
      d. Swelling.
      e. Dystrophic changes.
  2. Causes include:
      a. Previous trauma/injury.
      b. Arthritis.
      c. Tendinitis.
      d. Infection.
      e. Tumor.
      f. Myocardial infarction (MI).
      g. Herpes zoster
      h. Herniated lumbar disk.
  3. Sensitivity of bone scan—96%; specificity—97%.
  4. Findings.
      a. Diffusely increased blood flow to involved area.
      b. Increased blood pool compared with opposite side.
      c. Delayed images—diffusely increased periarticular uptake in involved extremity.
      d. Positive bone scans often return to normal following corticosteroid therapy.

M. Heterotopic ossification (HO).
  1. Associated with paraplegia and quadriplegia. Approximately 25% of patients develop HO following spinal cord injury.
  2. Many present with evidence of acute inflammation that can be

confused with deep venous thrombosis (DVT) or infection. Can eventually lead to joint ankylosis and immobility.
3. About 4 to 10 weeks after injury, HO may begin and will progress for 6 to 18 months.
4. Bone scan more sensitive early than plain film. In addition, useful for following maturity.
5. Findings—Increased activity in soft tissues on delayed images.
6. Determining maturity.
   a. Possible decrease in recurrence if HO surgically removed when mature.
   b. Maturity can be determined with serial bone scans when activity decreases then plateaus.
   c. Development of uptake on marrow scan also evidence of maturity.
N. Arthritides.
1. Degenerative joint disease.
   a. Destruction of cartilage results in abnormal stress on adjacent bone. This causes osteogenesis, accounting for increased uptake on bone scan.
   b. In addition, increased synovial capillary permeability/joint effusion may allow agents to diffuse across synovial membrane.
   c. Finally, bone agent may bind to proteins within joint fluid.
   d. Most common locations are:
      (1) Hands.
      (2) Feet.
      (3) Hips.
      (4) Knees.
      (5) SI joints.
      (6) Shoulders.
2. Rheumatoid arthritis.
   a. Rheumatoid arthritis and related diseases (psoriatic arthritis, ankylosis spondylitis, Reiter's syndrome) result in inflammation of synovial membrane and hypervascularity. Increased flow and bone remodeling account for increased uptake on bone scan.
   b. Rheumatoid arthritis (RA) findings:
      (1) Increased flow.
      (2) Symmetrical increased uptake on delayed views.
      (3) Primary distribution involves:
         (a) Hands.
         (b) Feet.
         (c) Knees.

  (d) Cervical spine.

 (4) In hands involvement primarily:

  (a) Metacarpal/phalangeal.

  (b) Proximal interphalangeal.

 c. Scan more sensitive than plain films or clinical examinations.

3. Pseudarthrosis.

 a. False joint at area of fusion.

 b. Findings.

  (a) Increased uptake at point of pseudarthrosis.

  (2) May see cold area as a result of fibrous tissue.

  (3) Note: Increased uptake may persist at least 6 months following spinal fusion because of postsurgical changes.

SUGGESTED READINGS

Alazraki N: Diagnosing prosthetic joint infection (editorial). *J Nucl Med* 1990; 31:1955-1957.

Alazraki N: Musculoskeletal imaging. In Taylor AT, Datz FL (eds): *Clinical practice of nuclear medicine.* Churchill Livingstone, New York, 1991, pp 379-431.

Alazraki N: Radionuclide techniques in radiography of the musculoskeletal system. In Resnick D, Niwayama G (eds): *Diagnosis of bone and joint disorders.* W B Saunders, Philadelphia, 1981, pp 639-679.

Ali A, Tetalman MR, Fordham EW, et al: Distribution of hypertrophic pulmonary osteoarthropathy. *AJR* 1980; 134:771-780.

Bitran JD, Bekerman C, Desser RK: The predictive value of serial bone scans in assessing response to chemotherapy in advanced breast cancer. *Cancer* 1980; 45:1562-1568.

Butzelaar RMJM, Van Dongen JA, DeGraff PW, et al: Bone scintigraphy in patients with operable breast cancer stages I and II: Final conclusion after five-year followup. *Eur J Cancer Clin Oncol* 1984; 20:877-880.

Coleman RE, Mashter G, Whitaker KB, et al: Bone scan flare predicts successful systemic therapy for bone metastases. *J Nucl Med* 1988; 29:1354-1359.

Collier BD, Carrera GF, Johnson RP, et al: Detection of femoral head avascular necrosis in adults by SPECT. *J Nucl Med* 1985; 26:979-987.

Collier BD, Carrera GF, Messer EJ, et al: Internal derangement of the temporomandibular joint: Detection by single-photon emission computed tomography. *Radiology* 1983; 149:557-561.

Corcoran RJ, Thrall JH, Kyle RW, et al: Solitary abnormalities in bone scans of patients with extraosseous malignancies. *Radiology* 1976; 121:663-667.

Datz FL: Radionuclide imaging of joint inflammation in the '90s. *J Nucl Med* 1990; 31:684-687.

Gelman MI, Coleman RE, Stevens, PM, et al: Radiography, radionuclide imaging, and arthrography in the evaluation of total hip and knee replacement. *Radiology* 1978; 128:667-682.

Ghaed N, Thrall JH, Pinsky SM, et al: Detection of extraosseous metastases from osteosarcoma with ^{99m}Tc-polyphosphate bone scanning. *Radiology* 1974; 112:373-375.

Harcke HT: Bone imaging in infants and children: A review. *J Nucl Med* 1978; 19:324-329.

Helms CA: Osteoid osteoma: the double density sign. *Clin Orthop* 1987; 222:167-173.

Holder LE, Mackinnon SE: Reflex sympathetic dystrophy in the hands: Clinical and scintigraphic critera. *Radiology* 1984; 152:517-522.

Holder LE, Michael RH: The specific scintigraphic pattern of "shin splints in the lower leg": Concise communication. *J Nucl Med* 1984; 25:865-869.

Hortobagyi GN, Libshitz HI, Seabold JE: Osseous metastases of breast cancer: Clinical, biochemical, radiographic, and scintigraphic evaluation of response to therapy. *Cancer* 1984; 53:577-582.

Jackson DW, Wiltse LL, Dingeman RD, et al: Stress reactions involving the pars interarticularis in young athletes. *Am J Sports Med* 1981; 9:304-312.

Jacobson AF, Stomper PC, Cronin EB, et al: Bone scans with one-two abnormalities in cancer patients with no known metastates: Reliability of interpretation of initial correlative radiographs. *Radiology* 1990; 174:503-507.

Levenson RM, Sauerbrunn BJL, Bates HR, et al: Comparative value of bone scintigraphy and radiography in monitoring tumor response in systemically treated prostatic carcinoma. *Radiology* 1983; 146:513-518.

Lund F, Smith PH, Suciu S, et al. Do bone scans predict prognosis in prostatic cancer? A report of the EORTC protocol 30762. *Br J Urol* 1984; 56:58-63.

Manier SM, van Nostrand D: From "hot spots" to "superscan." *Clin Nucl Med* 1983; 8:624-625.

Martin P: Bone scanning of trauma and benign conditions. In Freeman LM, Weissman HS (eds): *Nuclear medicine annual,* New York, Raven, 1982, pp 81-118.

Martin P: Bone scintigraphy in the diagnosis and management of traumatic injury. *Semin Nucl Med* 1983; 13:104-122.

Maurer AH, Chen DCP, Camargo EE, et al: Utility of three-phase skeletal scintigraphy in suspected osteomyelitis: Concise communication. *J Nucl Med* 1981; 22:941-949.

McAfee JG: Radionuclide imaging in metabolic and systemic skeletal diseases. *Semin Nucl Med* 1987; 16:344-349.

McKillop JH, Etcubanas E, Goris MI: The indications for and limitations of bone scintigraphy in osteogenic sarcoma: A review of 55 patients. *Cancer* 1981; 48:1133-1138.

McNeil BJ: Value of bone scanning in neoplastic disease. *Semin Nucl Med* 1984; 14:277-286.

Orzel JA, Rudd TG: Heterotopic bone formation: Clinical, laboratory, and imaging correlation. *J Nucl Med* 1985; 26:125-132.

Park HM, Wheat LJ, Siddiqui AR, et al: Scintigraphic evaluation of diabetic osteomyelitis. Concise communication. *J Nucl Med* 1982; 23:569-573.

Pollen JJ, Witztum KF, Ashburn WI: The flare phenomenon on radionuclide bone scan in metastatic prostate cancer. *AJR* 1984; 142:773-776.

Rosen PR, Murphy KG: Bone scintigraphy in the initial staging of patients with renal cell carcinoma: Concise communication. *J Nucl Med* 1984; 25: 289-291.

Rossleigh MA, Lovegrove FTA, Reynolds, PM, et al: Serial bone scans in the assessment of response to therapy in advanced breast carinoma. *Clin Nucl Med* 1982; 7:397-402.

Rupani, HD, Holder LE, Espinola DA, et al: Three-phase radionuclide bone imaging in sports medicine. *Radiology* 1985; 156:187-196.

Schauwerker DS: Osteomyelitis: Diagnosis with ^{111}In-labeled leukocytes. *Radiology* 1989; 171:141-146.

Smith FW, Gilday DL: Scintigraphic appearances of osteoid osteoma. *Radiology* 1980; 137:191-195.

Smith FW, Gukdat, DI, Ash JM, et al: Primary neuroblastoma uptake of [99m]technetium methylene disphosphate. *Radiology* 1980; 137:501-504.

Sty JR, Starshak RJ: The role of bone scintigraphy in the evaluation of the suspected abused child. *Radiology* 1983; 146:369-375.

Tanaka T, Rossier AB, Hussey RW, et al: Quantitative assessment of para-osteoarthropathy and its maturation on serial radionuclide bone images. *Radiology* 1977; 123:217-221.

Todd BD, Godfrey LW, Bodley RN: Intraoperative radioactive localization of an osteoid osteoma: A useful variation in technique. *Br J Radiol* 1989; 62:187-189.

4

Pulmonary Imaging

PULMONARY SYSTEM
Anatomy

I. Vascular system.
  A. Lungs divided into lobes and discrete bronchopulmonary segments, each with its own artery and vein (and bronchus). Pulmonary emboli occlude vessels supplying, and within, these segments. Therefore, PE associated with segmental defects, whereas other diseases usually affect flow in a nonsegmental manner.
  B. In adults, 280 billion pulmonary arterioles small enough to trap 20- to 40-μ particles used for perfusion scanning. In newborns, significantly smaller numbers of pulmonary alveoli and arterioles. Number increases rapidly over first 12 months of life, then more gradually, until adult numbers reached at age 8 years. Thus, smaller number of radioactive particles must be used to scan young children.

II. Airways.
  A. Trachea → main stem bronchi → segmental bronchi → bronchioles → terminal bronchioles → alveolar ducts → alveolar sacs → alveoli.
  B. Cartilage supports airway from the trachea to bronchioles. More distally, support is from smooth muscle only.
  C. In addition to airflow through above pathway, gas can be exchanged through:
    1. Pores of Kohn—connect neighboring alveoli.
    2. Canals of Lambert—connect respiratory bronchioles and alveolar ducts.
    3. These indirect connections allow collateral air drift. Air can enter part of lung where branches, segmental or smaller, are obstructed, preventing atelectasis. They also allow xenon during equilibrium or rebreathing phase of ventilation study to reach portions of lung that are not ventilated through normal channels such as in chronic obstructive pulmonary disease (COPD).

D. Alveoli—250 million to 300 million in adults.
   1. Lined by alveolar type I and II cells. Type II cells, found at corners of alveoli, secrete surfactant.

Physiology

I. Blood flow.
   A. Gravity causes uneven regional distribution of blood flow. In upright position, 3 to 5 times greater blood flow per unit volume in lower lung fields compared with upper. In any region of lung, blood flow is determined by balance between alveolar pressure, pulmonary arterial pressure, pulmonary venous pressure, and interstitial pressure.
   B. In upper parts of upright lung, alveolar pressure exceeds pulmonary arterial pressure, causing capillaries to collapse. Blood passes through only at peaks of pulmonary arterial pressure. More inferiorly, pulmonary arterial pressure exceeds alveolar pressure with flow occurring continuously. This accounts for apex-to-basilar gradient.
II. Ventilation.
   A. Alveolar ventilation is due to changes in intrapleural pressure (the pressure in potential space between visceral and parietal pleura).
   B. Inspiration.
      1. Intercostal muscles and diaphragm contract, expanding the chest.
      2. This causes intrapleural pressure to fall. Fall in pressure overcomes elastic recoil forces of the lung and resistance to airflow in bronchi.
   C. Expiration.
      1. Primarily caused by elastic recoil. Recoil made up of:
         a. Surface tension of alveoli—most important component.
         b. Connective tissue supporting lungs (collagen and elastic fibers).
   D. Like perfusion, ventilation not uniform in the lung because of gravity.
      1. Gravity causes intrapleural pressure to be less in more dependent regions of lung—the bases. This means transpulmonary pressure (force between alveoli and pleura) is greater at apex of lung than at base. Thus, alveoli in apices more expanded at expiration than alveoli in bases.
         a. This puts alveoli in bases on steep proportion of pressure-volume curve, meaning there is greater change in volume of basilar alveoli compared with apical alveoli for the same

change in intrapulmonary pressure. Thus, gas exchange increases from apex to base.

III. Ventilation—perfusion ratio.
  A. Blood flow—increases from 3- to 5-fold apex to base.
  B. Ventilation increases 1.5- to 2.0-fold from apex to base.
  C. Thus, ventilation-perfusion (VP) ratio falls from 2 to 3 in the apices to 0.6 at base.
  D. VP ratio is more important determinant of concentration of O_2 and CO_2 in the pulmonary capillary blood than the absolute amount of ventilation or perfusion. As ratio falls, O_2 content falls.
    1. Oxygen—because of shape of O_2-hemoglobin dissociation curve, a region with high VP ratio cannot correct for an area with low ratio.
    2. CO_2—CO_2-blood association curve less flat over working range; therefore, CO_2 can be corrected by areas of lung with high VP ratios.
IV. Pathophysiology.
  A. Blood flow—many diseases other than pulmonary emboli decrease pulmonary blood flow.
    1. Emphysema—alveolar capillary bed destroyed in some areas, especially those affected by bullous disease.
    2. Chronic bronchitis/asthma—bronchoconstriction causes hypoxia. Homeostatic mechanisms, in attempt to maintain symmetry of distribution of ventilation and perfusion, cause reflex pulmonary arteriolar constriction, diminishing flow.
  B. Ventilation.
    1. Emphysema.
      a. Dilatation and destruction of alveoli occur with loss of alveolar surface area. Elastic recoil forces diminished. Support of small airways by neighboring alveoli seriously weakened, leading to narrowing and irregularity. Air flow rates and gas exchange hampered due to:
      (1) Increase in airway resistance.
      (2) Loss of driving force for expiration.
      (3) Reduced alveolar surface area in capillary bed.
    2. Chronic bronchitis.
      a. Increase in mucous glands, excessive secretions, thickening of mucosa, irregular narrowing of airways occurs. Infection may help induce inflammation of bronchial walls and bronchospasm. Changes take place first in small airways; because these contribute so little to airway resistance, routine pulmonary function tests may be normal in young cigarette smokers.

3. Bonchoconstriction in PE.
   a. Decreased perfusion rarely causes reflex bronchoconstriction. In experimental animals, only 1.5% of emboli induced reflux bronchoconstriction. When it occurred, it was transient, lasting only a few hours. Reports of persons with pulmonary emboli causing bronchoconstriction (and therefore retention on ventilation scan), i.e., ventilation-perfusion (V/Q) match, have been rare.

Radiopharmaceuticals

I. Perfusion agents.
   A. Macroaggregated albumin (MAA).
      1. Labeled with ^{99m}Tc.
      2. Prepared by denaturing human serum albumin with heat.
      3. 90% of particles are between 5 to 90 μ; majority are in the 10- to 40-μ range.
      4. Biologic half-life—2 to 9 hours. Leaves lungs by being broken down into smaller particles that enter general circulation and are removed by reticuloendothelial system of liver and spleen.
   B. Human albumin microspheres (HAM).
      1. Labeled with ^{99m}Tc.
      2. Produced by agitating human serum albumin in heated vegetable oil, forming spherically shaped particles. These passed through sieve to produce desired size.
      3. Size—10- to 45-μ diameter. Generally, microspheres show less variation in size than MAA.
      4. Biologic half-life—7 hours—longer than MAA. Unlike MAA, technetium leaches off HAM and enters circulation as free pertechnetate. Thus, one sees gastrointestinal (GI) tract and genitourinary (GU) activity after HAM scan rather than reticuloendothelial system.
      5. Greater number of reports of allergic reactions with microspheres compared with MAA.
   C. Macroaggregated albumin or human albumin microspheres.
      1. Minimum number of particles necessary to obtain even distribution of radioactivity in vascular bed is 60,000; therefore, 100,000 particles reasonable number to use.
      2. With instant kits, approximately 500,000 particles labeled (MAA) unless steps taken to reduce numbers.
      3. With 200,000 to 500,000 particles, approximately 1 vessel per 1,000 will be blocked in adults; thus, safety factor large.
      4. Those in whom number of particles should be reduced include:
         a. Children.

      b. Patients with severe pulmonary hypertension.

      c. Patients with right-to-left shunt.

II. Ventilation.

  A. Xenon 133.

    1. Most commonly used agent.

    2. Half-life—5.3 days.

    3. Decays by beta minus.

    4. Ventilation scan must be performed before perfusion scan because of lower energy of ^{133}Xe (81 keV) compared with technetium used to label lung perfusion agents (140 keV). Downscatter of activity from technetium into xenon window interferes with interpetation of ventilation scan.

    5. Disposal by trapping exhaled xenon gas and letting it decay.

  B. Xenon 127.

    1. Cyclotron produced.

    2. Decays by electron capture.

    3. Half-life—36.4 days.

    4. 172- and 203-keV photon; therefore, ventilation scan can be performed *after* perfusion.

      a. Allows cost saving in patients with normal perfusion scan.

      b. Ventilation scan can be performed in the projection that best shows any defects seen on perfusion scan.

    5. Problems.

      a. More expensive than ^{133}Xe.

      b. Higher energy requires more shielding of ventilator.

      c. Longer half-life and higher energy makes storage of xenon 127, as means of disposal, difficult.

      d. Reduced availability from manufacturer.

  C. Krypton 81m.

    1. Decays by isomeric transition.

    2. 13-second half-life.

    3. 190-keV photon.

    4. Due to short half-life, must be breathed directly from generator (rubidium 81m parent with 4.7-hour half-life).

    5. Allows ventilation studies to be performed after perfusion scan. Due to short half-life, only equilibrium can be obtained.

    6. Disadvantages.

      a. Occasional cases have been found in which minor ventilatory abnormalities occurred in regions of pulmonary embolism. Agreement with ^{133}Xe approximately 90%.

      b. Short half-life of parent means generator must be ordered frequently.

　　c. Expensive.
D. Aerosols.
　　1. Can tag with technetium, indium 111, indium 113m, etc.
　　2. Usual material is colloid or diethylene-triamine pentaacetic acid (DPTA).
　　3. Aerosol produced by nebulizer with a settling bag (or similar device) to trap large particles. Connected to non-rebreathing valve. Patient breathes material over 2- to 4-minute time span.
　　4. Site of deposition of particles is dependent on size. Larger particles (2 to 5 μ) deposit centrally in posterior pharynx and trachea. Poor peripheral penetration.
　　5. Particle of 0.5 μ and less produce superior peripheral penetration.
　　6. If labeled with indium 111 or 113m, may be performed after perfusion study due to the higher energy levels of these nuclides compared with technetium.
　　　　a. Alternatively, small dose of MAA can be used for perfusion scan (0.5 mCi) and large dose of technetium (30 mCi) can be aerosolized. Since approximately 10% of material ends up in patient's lungs, approximately 6 times greater dose of technetium DTPA (3 mCi) will be present than MAA, allowing the determination of fill in of ventilation in areas of perfusion defects.

Technique

I. Ventilation (^{133}Xe).
　A. Patient positioned upright with camera posterior.
　B. 15 to 20 mCi ^{133}Xe injected into the intake port as patient takes maximum inspiration.
　C. 100-K count single breath image obtained.
　D. Patient rebreathes xenon in closed spirometer system for 4 minutes. Rebreathing necessary to allow xenon to enter abnormal lung zones via collateral air drift.
　E. 300-K count equilibrium image obtained during or at end of equilibrium.
　F. Valves readjusted so patient breathes room air, washing out xenon.
　G. Washout images obtained at 30 to 60 second intervals for approximately 6 minutes.
　H. After first washout images, right and left posterior obliques can be performed. These better localize abnormal zones of xenon ventilation showing their anteroposterior location.
II. Perfusion.

A. Before injection, syringe should be shaken to resuspend particles.
B. Patient injected in supine position. This reduces apical-to-basal activity gradient.
C. Imaging performed immediately after injection.
D. With large-field-of-view camera, anterior, posterior, both laterals, and both anterior and posterior obliques obtained. Posterior view obtained for 500,000 counts; remainder of images collected for same time.

Normal Scan

I. Ventilation.
  A. Xenon 133 and 127.
    1. Two lungs appear almost as mirror images.
    2. Costophrenic angles are not as well seen as with MAA.
    3. Unlike perfusion, heart causes almost no defect. This due to low energy of xenon, so that anterior activity accounts for few counts in image compared with technetium scan. Note that ^{127}Xe shows more prominent heart defects.
    4. Washout—lower lung fields empty more quickly than upper regions. Lung activity usually gone by 3 minutes. Occasional patient shows slightly longer retention.
  B. Krypton 81.
    1. Similar to xenon equilibrium image. Trachea often faintly seen.
  C. Aerosols.
    1. Similar to perfusion scans.
    2. Often multiple focal hot spots representing deposition of aerosol in pharynx, trachea, and bronchi; swallowed material seen in stomach.
    3. If patient hyperventilates during study, there is increased central deposition that clears on delayed images.
    4. Asymptomatic cigarette smokers may show increased irregular central deposition.
II. Perfusion.
  A. MAA or HAM.
    1. Posterior view.
      a. Smooth outline with sharper costophrenic angles than seen on ventilation scan.
      b. Heart may make defect in left medial border, especially if cardiomegaly present.
      c. Hila and aortic knob may also cause defects along medial border.
    2. Anterior view.

      a. Prominent heart defect.

      b. In women, breasts may cause diffuse decreased activity in lung bases.

  3. Lateral views.

      a. Central, circular, or sunburst defects seen because of hila.

      b. Left lateral view shows concave defect resulting from heart. This may be faintly seen on right lateral as well, due to shine-through from opposite lung (20% to 30% of counts on lateral view come from oppostie lung). Note that heart defect is never triangular. If this shape is seen, it indicates lingular abnormality.

      c. Shoulders cause decreased activity in upper lung fields.

  4. Anterior oblique views.

      a. Excellent for evaluating lingual and right middle lobe.

      b. Costophrenic angles seen much more distinctly than on other views.

      c. Defects as a result of hila commonly seen.

  5. Posterior oblique (PO) views.

      a. Left PO—heart makes concave defect in anterolateral border.

      b. Prominent defects often present in upper posterior lung field due to overlying scapula and musculature. Can be very distinct and simulate a perfusion defect. The fact that this defect is not well seen on other views helps differentiate it from a true abnormality.

  6. Normal variants.

      a. Decreased activity in right apex.

      b. Decreased perfusion in azygos lobe.

      c. Obese patients—small lung volumes with blunted or even absent costophrenic angles that appear rounded upward.

Abnormal Scans

  I. Ventilation.

    A. Single breath image.

      1. Areas of decreased activity. These represent defects in regional ventilation—areas not normally ventilated well with tidal breathing.

      2. 67% of perfusion defects resulting from COPD detected on these images. Washout images are more sensitive. However, 7% of abnormalities missed on washout are present on single breath images.

    B. Equilibrium.

      1. Areas of decreased activity—indicate that total lung volume is not ventilated.

C. Washout images.
  1. Rebreathing allows xenon to reach areas of obstructed lung due to collateral air drift.
  2. Areas of obstructive lung disease show up as hot spots representing retained xenon.
  3. Most sensitive part of the ventilation scan for detecting areas of abnormal ventilation. Xenon/background ratio of negative defect on single breath image can never be greater than 1. Contrast of lesions showing up as hot spots on washout images can be many times this.
  4. Sensitivity and specificity of washout images vary with criteria. Three minutes commonly used as cutoff, giving acceptable sensitivity—83% and specificity—85%.
  5. Note that with low-energy photon of ^{133}Xe, areas of retention in anterior lung segments will not be as well detected as those of posterior segments.

II. Perfusion scans
  A. Areas of decreased activity.
  B. Best if defect confirmed in multiple views.
  C. Hot spots usually due to drawing back blood forming radioactive clots in the syringe and reinjecting into patient. May be seen rarely when injecting through vein involved with thrombophlebitis.

III. Pulmonary embolism.
  A. Clinical.
  1. Clinical diagnosis often difficult. Signs and symptoms nonspecific and may be absent.
  2. Classic triad—infrequently seen:
    a. Hemoptysis.
    b. Thrombophlebitis.
    c. Pleural friction rub.
  3. Most common symptoms.
    a. Dyspnea (86%).
    b. Cough (70%).
    c. Pleuritic chest pain (58%).
  4. Findings.
    a. Tachypnea.
    b. Tachycardia.
    c. Accentuation of pulmonic component of S2.
    d. Rales.
  5. Some studies indicate clinical diagnosis of PE correct in only 25% to 45% of patients.
  B. Laboratory findings.

1. Blood gases—decreased.
2. Electrocardiogram (ECG)—usually normal.
   a. If abnormal—evidence of right ventricular (RV) strain.
3. Chest x-ray.
   a. May be normal.
   b. Often nonspecific findings present such as:
      (1) Atelectasis.
      (2) Pleural effusion.
      (3) Elevated hemidiaphragm.
   c. Infarction (i.e., infiltrate) present in less than 10%.
   d. Oligemia—rarely seen.
C. Pulmonary angiography.
   1. Good sensitivity, excellent specificity.
   2. Invasive.
   3. Expensive.
   4. Associated with morbidity and mortality (although low).
IV. Findings of PE on V/Q scan.
   A. Perfusion scan.
      1. Pulmonary emboli defects are classically:
         a. Segmental—since blood flow corresponds to segmental anatomy of lung. May involve entire lobe, segment, or portion of segment (subsegmental). Occasionally, entire lung involved.
            (1) In study of patients with angiographically proven pulmonary emboli, 75% or more of individual emboli caused segmental defects. Remainder were more patchy, nonsegmental defects.
         b. Multiple.
            (1) As thrombus passes through right side of the heart, it breaks into fragments. Angiographic studies indicate average patient with pulmonary emboli has 11 emboli fragments. Approximately 20% to 25% of these fragments will not produce enough effect on blood flow to be detectable (or involve vessels too small to be detected). Large number of fragments ensure high sensitivity of perfusion scan.
            (2) Of experimental emboli that completely occlude 2.0 mm or larger vessels, 97% detected.
            (3) Even in smaller vessels, 66% detected.
            (4) Those causing partial defect, however, detected much less frequently, approximatley 25%.
         c. Peripheral.
            (1) Stripe sign—if stripe of activity seen, makes pul-

monary emboli unlikely, since pulmonary emboli are usually pleural based. Defect more likely due to chronic obstructive pulmonary disease (COPD), etc.

    (2) Shrunken lung sign—occasionally multiple, very small emboli lodge peripherally, causing lung to appear smaller than normal.

    (3) Fissure sign—if tiny emboli lodge along pleural surface that partly forms fissures, a linear defect, similar to pleural fluid, will be present. Fortunately, chances of seeing this sign (or shrunken lung sign) without other perfusion defects more recognizable as pulmonary emboli, are rare.

  d. Wedge-shaped.

  e. Due to anatomy of blood supply, somewhat of a predilection for lower lobes.

  f. Perfusion defects due to COPD are:

    (1) Nonsegmental—80%.

    (2) Often involve upper lobes even in absence of significant lower lobe defects.

    (3) Stripe sign often present.

B. Ventilation scan.

  1. Pulmonary embolism.

    a. V/Q mismatch, i.e., normal ventilation in area of diminished perfusion.

    b. Reflex bronchospasm.

      (1) 1.5% of experimental emboli in dogs result in bronchoconstriction.

      (2) When occurs is transient, lasting less than 4 to 8 hours.

      (3) Only few isolated cases reported in humans.

  2. Chronic obstructive pulmonary disease.

    a. V/Q match; i.e., abnormal ventilation in area of perfusion defect.

  3. Ventilation scan alters diagnosis in as many as 40% of patients, primarily reducing probability of PE from high to low. Specificity in COPD patients, combining V and Q scans, has been as high as 91%.

  4. In patients with severe and diffuse COPD in whom diffuse retention present (greater than one half of the lungs) you cannot match a specific perfusion defect to specific local area of retention. Presence of perfusion defects due to COPD *and* superimposed emboli *cannot* be reliably excluded.

V. Interpretation schemes for PE.

Table 4-1   Biello Scheme for Interpretation of V/Q Imaging

Interpretation	Pattern	Pulmonary Embolism Frequency (%)
Normal Probability of pulmonary embolism	Normal perfusion	0
Low	Small V/Q mismatches	0
	Focal V/Q matches with no corresponding radiographic abnormalities	4.8
	Perfusion defects substantially smaller than radiographic abnormalities	7.7
Intermediate	Diffuse, severe airway obstruction	20
	Matched perfusion defects and radiographic abnormalities	27
	Single moderate V/Q mismatch without corresponding radiographic abnormality	33
High	Perfusion defects substantially larger than radiographic abnormalities ≥1 large, or ≥2* moderate-sized V/Q mismatches with no corresponding radiographic abnormalities	87
		92

*Many nuclear medicine physicians categorize single mismatched defects, regardless of size, as intermediate.

A. No patterns on V/Q scanning that are diagnostic or exclusive of pulmonary embolism (except a normal scan) based on angiographic findings in patients. For this reason, V/Q scans usually read as normal, low, intermediate (indeterminate), or high probability.

B. Biello criteria.
   1. Widely used scheme. Developed by retrospectively reviewing V/Q scan appearance and correlating with pulmonary angiogram results.
   2. Perfusion scan defects are sized.
      a. Defect less than 25% of bronchopulmonary segment—small.
      b. 25% to 75%—moderate.
      c. >75%—large.
   3. Number in each size category totaled.
   4. Ventilation scan reviewed to determine if V/Q match or mismatch present.
   5. See Table 4-1 for category. Percentage in chart based on

Table 4-2   Indeterminate Lung Scintigrams (Comparison With Pulmonary Angiography)

Size of Perfusion Defect Compared With Radiographic Abnormality	Number of Patients	Pulmonary Embolism (%)
Smaller	14	7
Equal	77	26
Larger		
V/P mismatch	18	89
V/P match	2	0
Total	111	33

author's population. Does *not* take prior probability (i.e., degree of clinical suspicion of pulmonary emboli prior to study) into account.

6. Note if patient has moderate to severe COPD with diffuse xenon retention; categorize as intermediate. Note above scheme assumes no infiltrates present on chest x-ray.

C. Modification on Biello's criteria.
1. Many categorize solitary large defects as intermediate probability.

D. Application of Biello's criteria with infiltrates on chest film.
1. Helpful in differentiating pneumonia and other nonembolic causes of infiltrates from pulmonary infarct due to pulmonary emboli.
2. Done by comparing size of perfusion defect on scan with size of infiltrate on chest x-ray (Table 4-2).
   a. Perfusion defect significantly larger than x-ray infiltrate—high probability.
   b. Perfusion defect smaller than x-ray infiltrate—low probability.
   c. Defect and infiltrate same size—intermediate (indeterminate) probability.
3. Pleural effusions.
   a. Perfusion defect equal in size to pleural effusion on chest x-ray, and no other perfusion defects except small defects—low probability of pulmonary emboli. Note: This rule is somewhat controversial.

E. PIOPED criteria.
1. PIOPED = *P*rospective *I*nvestigation *O*f *P*ulmonary *E*mbolism *D*iagnosis.

Table 4-3   PIOPED Central Scan Intepretation Categories and Criteria

Category	Criteria
High probability	Two or more large (>75% of a segment) segmental perfusion defects without corresponding ventilation or radiographic abnormalities, or substantially larger than either matching ventilation or chest radiographic abnormalities Two or more moderate segmental (>25% and <75% of a segment) perfusion defects without matching ventilation or chest radiographic abnormalities and one large segmental deficit Four or more moderate subsegmental perfusion defects without ventilation or chest radiographic abnormalities
Intermediate probability (indeterminate)	Not falling into normal, very low, low, or high-probability categories Borderline high, borderline low Difficult to categorize as low or high
Low probability	Nonsegmental perfusion defects, e.g., very small effusion causing blunting of the costophrenic angle (cardiomegaly; enlarged aorta, hila, and mediastinum; and elevated diaphragm) Single moderate mismatched segmental perfusion defect with normal chest radiograph Any perfusion defect with a substantially *larger* chest radiographic abnormality

2. A multi-institutional study of the sensitivity and specificity of V/Q scanning for pulmonary embolism.
3. A modification of the Biello criteria was developed to use in the study (Table 4-3).
4. Note that these criteria were developed *before* the study began; they are *not* the result of the study.
5. Studies of comparing the PIOPED criteria to Biello's criteria (and other interpretation schemes) have shown that Biello slightly outperforms PIOPED.

F. Prior probability.
1. Can be helpful to use prior probability (degree of clinical suspicion of pulmonary emboli before study) to help determine what to do with patients with abnormal V/Q scan. Can be especially helpful in determining who should have pulmonary angiogram to confirm or exclude pulmonary emboli.
2. Clinicians categorize clinical suspicion as low, average, or

Table 4-4   Probabilistic Estimates of Pulmonary Embolism in Three Clinical Situations Associated With Selected Scintigraphic Outcomes

Scan Pattern	Posterior Probabilities for Clinical Chances of Pulmonary Embolism		
	Low	Average	High
Indeterminate	0.04	0.13	0.47*
Many perfusion defects, no ventilation study			
Subsegmental	0.01	0.02	0.09
Segmental	0.10*	0.27*	0.68*
Lobar	0.26*	0.54*	0.87
Man perfusion defects, V/Q mismatch			
Lobar/segmental	0.54*	0.80	0.96
Subsegmental	0.01	0.03	0.17
Many perfusion defects, an V/Q match	0	0	0

*Probabilistic estimates in intermediate range.

high (Table 4-4). Gives probability of pulmonary emboli based on V/Q and clinical probabilities.

3. Example: If scan shows matching infiltrate and perfusion defect in size, scan technically indeterminate. However, if clinicians think pneumonia likely, patient has only 13% chance of pulmonary emboli, making a pulmonary angiogram necessary in most cases. Note that in patients with indeterminate scan and high clinical suspicion, only 47% have pulmonary emboli.

G. Recurrent pulmonary embolism.

1. 30% to 60% of patients receiving anticoagulants develop new perfusion defects. May be due to several phenomena:

a. Fragmentation of proximal emboli that shower more distal vessels.

b. Emboli may resolve at different rates (or vessels involved with emboli may relax at different rates). Causes changes in relative pulmonary resistance so particles may preferentially go to previous defect areas, making new defects in other areas.

c. Different rates of relaxation of vasoconstriction.

2. When diagnosing pulmonary emboli in patients with past history of pulmonary emboli, resolution varies. In young, healthy individuals, most resolution occurs in first few days,

with majority occurring by 10 days. In 3 months most resolution has occurred. In older patients with lung disease,
defects resolve more slowly and less completely.

   3. When comparing scan views (i.e., LPO), they will not be
exactly same, so defects may appear slightly more prominent. Unlikely patient would have pulmonary emboli in
same site as before. Look for defects in different areas.

H. Causes of V/Q mismatch other than acute pulmonary emboli.

   1. Past pulmonary emboli.

   2. Tumors such as bronchogenic carcinoma.

   3. Other emboli (air, talc, cotton fiber—drug addicts).

   4. Vasculitis.

   5. Radiation therapy.

I. Accuracy of V/Q scanning for PE.

   1. As noted above, PIOPED performed to determine accuracy
of V/Q scanning in pulmonary embolism.

   2. 933 patients prospectively studied.

   3. Angiographic incidence of PE (positive predictive value) for
each PIOPED classification:

     a. High probability—88%.

     b. Intermediate probability—33%.

     c. Low probability—12%.

     d. Normal—0%.

   4. Note similarity to Biello's retrospective study results.

VI. Chronic obstructive pulmonary disease (COPD).

A. Emphysema.

   1. Clinical.

     a. Caused primarily by cigarette smoking.

     b. More common in older patients.

   2. Pathophysiology.

     a. Dilatation and destruction of alveoli causes loss of alveo-
lar surface area and pulmonary capillary bed.

     b. Support of small airways by neighboring alveoli weak-
ened, leading to narrowing and irregularity of these small
airways. These changes lead to poor ventilation due to:

       (1) Increased airway resistance.

       (2) Loss of elastic recoil for expiration.

       (3) Reduced gas exchange.

   3. Findings.

     a. Ventilation.

       (1) Central lobular emphysema—predominantly lower
lobe disease.

       (2) Panlobular emphysema—diffuse involvement.

    (3) Usually ventilatory defects are patchy and nonsegmental. Degree of retention and distribution varies with severity. Discrete segmental lobar defects may occur.

    (4) Emphysematous bullae. Usually fail to fill during single breath or equilibrium.

    (5) Clearance of xenon correlates with forced expiratory volume (FEV_1).

    (6) Alpha$_1$-antitrypsin deficiency—most severe lower lobes. Symptomless heterozygotes usually show abnormalities as well.

  b. Perfusion.

    (1) Early, little effect.

    (2) Changes usually less than defects in ventilation.

    (3) 80% of perfusion defects patchy and nonsegmental; 15% to 20% segmental. Segmental defects accompanied by most severe derangements of regional ventilation.

B. Chronic bronchitis.

  1. Increase in mucus glands, thickening of mucosa, excessive secretions of mucus, irregular narrowing of airways.

  2. Earliest changes in small airways.

  3. Infections produce inflammation of bronchial walls and sometimes bronchospasm.

  4. These changes lead to:

    a. Increase in airway resistance.

    b. Hypoxic vasoconstriction.

    c. The matching of ventilation/blood flow is less accurate in chronic bronchitis than emphysema.

    d. Both chronic bronchitis and emphysema coexist in most patients, making it difficult to separate on scan.

C. Bronchial asthma.

  1. Background—airflow obstruction caused by bronchospasm, mucosal edema, and mucus plugging.

  2. Ventilation study.

    a. Single breath and washout abnormalities often more severe than accompanying perfusion defect.

  3. Perfusion.

    a. Subsegmental, segmental, and lobar perfusion defects indistinguishable from pulmonary emboli.

  4. Acute attack subsides, ventilation and perfusion improve, mimicking resolving pulmonary emboli.

  5. Between attacks some have normal scans; others, persistent abnormalities.

VII. Mucus plug syndrome.
  A. Background.
    1. Mucus plugs occur in quadriplegics and others who cannot clear secretions normally.
    2. Also occurs in those with thick viscous mucus—such as in cystic fibrosis.
    3. Airway obstruction causes local hypoxia and reflex vasoconstriction.
    4. Because of pores of Kohn, atelectasis may not occur to significant degree to be visible on chest x-ray examination.
  B. Ventilation.
    1. Shows significant retention.
  C. Perfusion.
    1. Like asthmatic, segmental defects mimic pulmonary embolism.
VIII. Lung carcinoma.
  A. Ventilation studies.
    1. Abnormal ventilation.
  B. Perfusion.
    1. Perfusion defects. Produce defects through mass effect, since derive blood supply from bronchial arteries.
      a. When involved vessels are at the hilum, segmental, lobar, or whole lung defects may be produced.
      b. Since endobronchial obstruction is usually less than extrabronchial spread, perfusion usually affected more significantly than ventilation.
  C. Foreign-body obstruction or tumor shows similar findings.
  D. Pneumonectomy evaluation.
    1. Quantitative V/Q performed. Percentage of perfusion and flow is calculated for each lung, then combined with patient's FEV_1. Values less than 0.8 to 1 are in high-risk group to develop pulmonary insufficiency postoperatively.
IX. Congestive heart failure.
  A. Ventilation.
    1. Usually normal.
    2. In patients with audible rales, bi-basilar retention may be seen. This is thought to be a result of edema of terminal bronchioles, causing impaired gas exchange.
  B. Perfusion.
    1. Interstitial pulmonary edema—perfusion scan normal or shows patchy nonsegmental defects. Only if patient in florid failure with alveolar edema will more prominent defects occur; however, these are usually nonsegmental.

2. Reversal of normal upper-to-lower lobe perfusion ratio. Due to vascular redistribution.
3. Fissure-sign—defect caused by pleural fluid.
X. Primary pulmonary hypertension.
  A. Background.
    1. For therapy, need to differentiate primary pulmonary hypertension (PPH) and thromboembolic pulmonary hypertension (TPH).
    2. Poor prognosis; average survival from time of onset, 3 years or less.
    3. Patients with TPH may be treated with vena caval interruption, anticoagulants, pulmonary thromboarterectomies.
    4. PPH treated with vasodilators.
  B. Primary pulmonary hypertension.
    1. Perfusion—normal or small subsegmental defects (i.e., low probability).
  C. Thromboembolic pulmonary hypertension.
    1. Ventilation—normal
    2. Perfusion—multiple segmental or lobar defects (i.e., high probability).
XI. Smoke inhalation.
  A. Background.
    1. One third of patients admitted to burn units have associated inhalation injury. Their mortality rate increases 2.5 times.
    2. Injury caused by toxic gases and small smoke particles that penetrate to distal airways. Causes edema of tracheobronchial mucosa. Eventually leads to atelectasis and infection.
  B. Laboratory.
    1. Chest x-ray examination usually normal during first few days.
    2. Accuracy of scan—92%.
  C. Technique.
    1. Procedure.
      a. 10 mCi of xenon dissolved in saline injected IV.
      b. 30-second images taken anteriorly over chest.
      c. Injected with 3 mCi ^{99m}Tc MAA.
      d. Multiple perfusion images obtained.
    2. Findings.
      a. Normal.
        (1) Xenon washes out by 120 seconds. No evidence of perfusion defects.
      b. Abnormal.
        (1) Focal retention. Diffuse retention rarely due to

smoke inhalation. Likely a result of decreased ventilation or COPD.

(2) Usually *not* associated with perfusion defect, but reason is unknown. Presence of perfusion defects with
matched retention raises likelihood of COPD.

(3) A common artifact is increased focal activity because
of a bubble of xenon coming out of solution and
remaining in the pulmonary artery. Central location
of bubble makes it recognizable.

SUGGESTED READINGS

Alderson PO, Biello DR, Gottschalk A, et al: Tc-99m DTPA aerosol and radioactive gases compared as adjuncts to perfusion scintigraphy in patients with suspected pulmonary embolism. *Radiology* 1984; 153:516-521.

Alderson PO, Biello DR, Khan AR, et al: Comparison of Xe-133 single breath
and washout images in scintigraphic diagnosis of pulmonary embolism. *Radiology* 1980; 137:481-486.

Adlerson PO, Biello DR, Sachariah KG, et al: Scintigraphic detection of pulmonary embolism in patients with obstructive pulmonary disease. *Radiology*
1981; 138:661-666.

Alderson PO, Line BR: Scintigraphic evaluation of regional pulmonary ventilation. *Semin Nucl Med* 1980; 10:218-242.

Alderson PO, Martin EC: Pulmonary embolism: Diagnosis with multiple imaging
modalities. *Radiology* 1987; 164:297-312.

Bedont RA, Datz FL: Lung scan perfusion defects limited to matching pleural
effusions: Low probability of pulmonary embolism. *AIR* 1985; 145:1155-1157.

Biello DR, Mattar AG, McKnight RC, et al: Interpretation of ventilation-perfusion studies in patients with suspected pulmonary embolism. *AJR* 1979;
133:1033-1037.

Biello DR, Mattar AG, Osei-Wusu A, et al: Interpretation of indeterminate lung
scintigrams. *Radiology* 1979; 133:189-194.

Datz FL: Lung imaging—ventilation/perfusion mismatch. In Taylor AT, Datz FL
(eds): *Gamuts in nuclear medicine,* ed 2. East Norwalk, Connecticut, Appleton
& Lange, 1987, pp 146-147.

Datz FL: Pulmonary Imaging. In Datz FL: *Clinical practice of nuclear medicine,*
New York, Churchill-Livingstone, 1991, pp 257-282.

Hayes, M, Taplin BF, Chopra SK, et al: Improved radioaerosol administration
system for routine inhalation lung imaging. *Radiology* 1979; 131:256-258.

Lee ME, Biello DR, Kumar B, et al: Clinical outcomes of patients with suspected
pulmonary embolism and "low probability" ventilation perfusion scintigrams.
Radiology 1985; 156:497-500.

Lull RJ, Anderson JH, Telepak RJ, et al: Radionuclide imaging in the assessment
of lung injury. *Semin Nucl Med* 1980; 10:302-310.

Moser KM, Longo AM, Ashburn WL, et al: Spurious scintiphotographic recurrence of pulmonary emboli, *Am J Med* 1973; 55:434-443.

Neumann RD, Sostman HD, Gottschalk A: Current status of ventilation-perfusion imaging *Semin Nucl Med* 1980; 10:198-217.

Osborne DR, Jaszcak RJ, Greer K, et al: Detection of pulmonary emboli in dogs: Comparison of single-photon emission computed tomography, gamma camera imaging and angiography. *Radiology* 1983; 146:493-498.

PIOPED Investigators: Value of ventilation/perfusion scan in acute pulmonary embolism: Results of the prospective investigation of pulmonary embolism diagnosis (PIOPED). *JAMA* 1990; 263:2753-2759.

Rosen JM, Biello DR, Siegel BA, et al: Kr-81m ventilation imaging: Clinical utility in suspected pulmonary embolism. *Radiology* 1985; 154:787-790.

Sostman HD, Gottschalk A: The stripe sign: A new sign for diagnosis of nonembolic defects on pulmonary perfusion scintigraphy. *Radiology* 1982; 142:737-741.

Sostman HD, Rapaport S, Gottschalk A, et al: Imaging of pulmonary embolism. *Investig Radiol* 1986; 21:443-454.

Strauss EB, Sostman HD, Gottschalk A: Radiographic parenchymal opacity, matching perfusion defect, and normal ventilation: A sign of pulmonary embolism? *Radiology* 1987; 163:505-506.

Sullivan DC, Coleman RE, Mills SR, et al: Lung scan interpretations: Effect of different observers and different criteria. *Radiology* 1983; 149:803-897.

Webber MM, Gomes AS, Roe D, et al: Comparison of Biello, McNeil, and PIOPED criteria for diagnosis of pulmonary emboli on lung scans. *AJR* 1990; 154:975-981.

5

Gastrointestinal and Hepatobiliary Imaging

LIVER-SPLEEN SCANNING
Anatomy

I. Liver
- A. One of largest organs in body. Weight 1,500 g. Covered by peritoneum except for superior surface. Diaphragm can make linear impressions on liver.
- B. Divided into four lobes.
    1. Right—80% of mass.
    2. Left—15% of mass.
    3. Caudate and quadrate lobes—5% of mass.
    4. Falciform ligament approximately divides liver into left and right lobes. The liver often has a notch at the superior and inferior margins of the ligament.
- C. Gallbladder—lies in fossa between right and quadrate lobes. Rarely intrahepatic.
- D. Renal fossa—created by right kidney in right lobe.
- E. Porta hepatis—depression on posterior central portion of the liver formed by hepatic artery, portal vein, and common bile duct.
- F. Blood supply.
    1. Portal vein. Formed by confluence of splenic and superior mesenteric vein. Accounts for 75% of liver blood flow.
    2. Hepatic artery accounts for remaining 25% of flow.
- G. Histology.
    1. Hepatocytes—vast majority of liver cells. Responsible for bile production.
    2. Kupffer's cells—line liver sinusoids. Remove cellular debris, bacteria, and other particulate matter, including radioactive colloids.

II. Spleen.
- A. Weight—165 g.
- B. Often associated with lobulations, notches, and clefts as result of spleen's fetal development.

C. Accessory spleen produced when some clusters of primordial spleen cells fail to fuse.
D. Blood supply.
 1. Splenic artery and vein—main supply and drainage.
 2. Vessels enter spleen through central indentation of visceral surface—hilum.
E. Histology—contains both pulp and venous sinusoids lined by reticuloendothelial system (RES) cells.

Physiology

I. Liver.
A. Hepatocytes responsible for clearing large number of substances and metabolizing them. Form bile.
B. Kupffer's cells responsible for phagocytosis. 95% of injected colloid particles cleared in a single pass. Factors that influence rate of phagocytosis by these cells include:
 1. Blood flow.
 2. RES cell function.
 3. Characteristics of particles.
  a. Number.
  b. Size.
  c. Charge.
  d. Presence of opsonins.
  e. Other physical characteristics.
II. Spleen.
A. Serves as reservoir.
B. Antibody production by splenic lymphocytes.
C. Phagocytizes senescent red cells, inclusions, small particles.
D. Percentage of colloids phagocytized by the spleen increases as particle size increases.
E. Normal distribution of injected colloids:
 1. 86% in RES of liver.
 2. 6% in spleen.
 3. 8% in RES of bone marrow.

Radiopharmaceuticals

I. Gold 198.
A. First radiocolloid used.
B. High radiation exposure.
II. Technetium 99m sulfur colloid.
A. Produced by reacting pertechnetate with sodium thiosulfate in an acidified solution.
B. Particle size—0.1 to 1.0 μm.

C. Most commonly used agent.
III. Technetium 99m albumin colloid.
   A. Particle size—0.2-1.0 μm.

Imaging Technique

I. Flow study.
   A. Use 5 to 6 mCi minimum.
   B. Imaging performed 2 to 3 seconds—multiformattor; two frames per second on computer for 60 seconds.
   C. 1-minute blood pool image can also be performed.
II. Static imaging.
   A. Large-field-of-view camera, parallel-hole all-purpose collimator, 20% window.
   B. 1 million counts or ID of 3,000 counts/sq cm.
   C. Anterior view with lead marker over costal margin and a size marker performed, followed by posterior, right/left laterals, right/left anterior obliques, and left posterior oblique.
III. SPECT imaging.
   A. Exact protocol varies with number of camera heads.
   B. Dual-headed camera.
      1. High-resolution, low energy parallel-hole collimator.
      2. 360 degree rotation.
      3. 128 × 128 matrix.
      4. 120 stops; 30 seconds/stop.

Normal Scan

I. Liver.
   A. Variable shape.
   B. Right lobe usually significantly larger than left. Thinning of left lobe can be mistaken for mass.
   C. Defects caused by gallbladder fossa, renal fossa.
   D. Central defect due to porta hepatis frequently seen.
   E. Occasionally vertical line of decreased activity present because of falciform ligament.
   F. Occasionally right lobe greatly elongated—Riedel's lobe.
   G. Breast attenuation in superior right lobe frequently seen in females on anterior and right lateral views.
   H. Size.
      1. Determined on the anterior view.
      2. 17 ± 2 cm maximum cephalocaudad length.
II. Spleen length.
   A. Determined on posterior view.
   B. Normal 10 ± 3 cm; 5 cm at birth. Up to age 16, L = 5.7 + 0.31 × A (A = age in years, L = length in centimeters).

Abnormal Findings

I. Early flow.
   A. Background.
      1. Seventy-five percent of liver perfusion from portal system. Liver normally not seen for 6 seconds after aortic activity.
      2. Malignant tumors in liver fed by hepatic artery. Seen as earlier flow. Hepatitis and other diffuse inflammatory diseases may show similar findings.
II. Increased flow.
   A. Focal hot spots seen in 50% of metastases, 90% hepatomas. (Figures for metastases from written reports; in our experience, number much less.)
   B. Hemangiomas.
      1. Usually do not show increased activity in hepatic angiogram. Best way to demonstrate increased blood pool activity in hemangiomas is with ^{99m}Tc labeled red blood cells.
III. Delayed/decreased flow.
   A. Causes.
      1. Congestive heart failure (CHF)—most common.
      2. Severe cirrhosis.
IV. Hepatomegaly.
   A. Most common abnormality on liver-spleen scan. More common in diffuse disease, although can occur in focal disease.
   B. With massive enlargement, likely causes:
      1. Fatty infiltration.
      2. Chronic passive congestion.
V. Splenomegaly.
   A. Nonspecific finding.
   B. With giant splenomegaly, consider:
      1. Chronic myelogenous leukemia.
      2. Myelofibrosis with myeloid metaplasia.
      3. Gaucher's disease.
      4. Malaria.
      5. Kala-azar.
VI. Shunting.
   A. Term describes greater activity in spleen than liver on posterior view, or increased bone marrow uptake.
   B. Pathophysiology.
      1. Changes in blood flow.
      2. Diminished liver uptake allowing more splenic and marrow uptake.
      3. Stimulation of the RES.

C. Specific causes include:
1. Hepatocellular dysfunction (hepatitis, cirrhosis).
2. Blood diseases (anemia, leukemia).
3. System infection.
4. Systemic tumor.
5. Diabetes.
6. CHF.
7. Ideopathic.

VII. Liver hot spots.
A. Rare.
B. Pathophysiology.
1. Increased perfusion:
a. Superior vena cava obstruction.
b. Budd-Chiari syndrome.
c. Tumors.
2. Increased number of Kupffer's cells:
a. Tumors.
C. Superior vena cava obstruction.
1. Background.
a. Most common cause of focal hot spot.
b. Lung cancer usual cause.
c. Colloid injected in arm shunted from obstructed superior vena cava through umbilical vein to left portal vein. Since umbilical vein supplies quadrate lobe, increased perfusion occurs producing focal hot spot.
d. With inferior vena cava obstruction, similar findings occur with foot injection.
D. Budd-Chiari syndrome.
1. Background.
a. Obstruction of hepatic vein because of tumor or clotting.
b. Vestigial connections between caudate lobe and inferior vena cava become patent, allowing venous drainage of this lobe. Improved perfusion produces hot spot.
c. Focal hot spot with decreased activity peripherally takes several months to develop. Acute Budd-Chiari syndrome presents as hepatomegaly and inhomgeneity only.
d. Radionuclide inferior vena cavagram helpful in diagnosis. Delayed flow is seen if disease process causing Budd-Chiari syndrome extends into vena cava.
E. Tumor.
1. Causes:
a. Focal nodular hyperplasia.
b. Hepatoma.

      2. Increased flow and increased number of RES cells contribute to increased activity.

VIII. Lung uptake.
- A. Technical.
  1. Aluminum contamination causes colloid clumping and lung embolization.
- B. Diseases.
  1. Hormone stimulation causes migration of macrophages into circulation. Lodge in precapillary arterioles and phagocytize sulfur colloid.
     - a. Cirrhosis.
     - b. Systemic tumor.
     - c. Systemic infection.

IX. Focal cold defects—liver.
- A. Causes.
  1. Metastases.
  2. Primary tumor—benign or malignant.
  3. Abscess.
  4. Cyst.

X. Cold defects in spleen.
  1. Causes.
     - a. Infarction.
     - b. Hematoma.
     - c. Abscess.
     - d. Cyst.
     - e. Hemangioma.

Focal Liver Disease

I. Metastatic disease.
- A. Background.
  1. Tumors that commonly metastasize to liver:
     - a. Breast.
     - b. Colon.
     - c. Lung.
     - d. Gastric.
     - e. Pancreas.
     - f. Cervical.
     - g. Uterine.
  2. Metastases most common cause of multiple cold defects on liver scan.
  3. Since metastases 20 times more common than primary hepatic tumors, metastases most common cause of solitary defects also.

B. Sensitivity—varies with primary and size of lesion.
   1. Colorectal tend to have larger, more discrete lesions—88%. Breast cancer, smaller more diffuse metastases, detect 67%.
   2. Varies by location.
      a. Lesion deep within liver may be missed.
      b. Lesions in left lobe also difficult to detect.
   3. Varies by type of imaging.
      a. Planar imaging—overall sensitivity 80% to 85%. Lesions less than 1.5 cm not detected. Those 1.5 to 2 cm, depends on location. Lesions greater than 2 cm usually detected.
      b. SPECT increases yield to approximately 90%.
C. Findings.
   1. Focal defect—most specific sign. Only 2% of metastases solitary at autopsy, therefore multiplicity good sign of metastases. As noted above, solitary lesions still likely to be metastasis, however.
   2. Inhomogeneity.
      a. Much lower specificity; however, must be considered in tumors such as breast.
   3. Hepatomegaly.
      a. Again, nonspecific.
      b. Not always present with metastases. Example: hepatomegaly present in only 50% of liver metastases in colorectal carcinoma.
   4. Increased flow to liver.
      a. Malignant tumors fed by hepatic artery, may be seen earlier than normal parenchyma. Appear as focal hot spots.
      b. Some data indicate 50% of metastases have this sign. In our experience, significantly less.
II. Primary malignant tumors.
  A. Hepatoma.
     1. Background.
        a. Most common primary malignant liver tumor.
        b. Majority associated with cirrhosis. Greater portion of patients with postnecrotic cirrhosis develop hepatoma; but, because alcoholic cirrhosis so much more common, greater absolute number associated with alcoholism.
     2. Findings.
        a. Solitary cold defect.
           (1) Up to two thirds of hepatomas appear this way.
           (2) Tumor grows rapidly, often quite large at presentation.

(3) Right lobe only or right and left lobes involved. Isolated left lobe involvement rare.
   b. Multiple cold defects. Approximately one sixth or more appear this way.
   c. Inhomogeneity/hepatomegaly only if diffuse involvement—one sixth.
   d. Focal hot spot—rare finding.
   e. Evidence of portal hypertension.
3. Other.
   a. Cholangiocarcinoma.
   b. Kupffer's cell carcinomas.
   c. No distinguishing characteristics for these tumors.

III. Benign tumors.
   A. Hepatic adenoma.
      1. Background.
         a. Second most common benign liver tumor.
         b. Occurs almost exclusively in women taking contraceptives.
         c. May present with massive hemorrhage.
         d. Pathologically consists of sheets of hepatocytes without bile ducts or Kupffer's cells.
      2. Findings.
         a. Solitary cold defect since adenomas usually lack Kupffer's cells. May be large.

IV. Focal nodular hyperplasia.
   A. Background.
      1. Consists of random collections of hepatocytes, bile ducts, and Kupffer's cells.
      2. Weak association with contraceptive use.
   B. Findings.
      1. Flow study—hypervascular.
      2. Appearance on delayed images depends on Kupffer's cell concentration.
         a. If number low—appear as cold defects—solitary (80%), or multiple (20%).
         b. If Kupffer's cell concentration equals that of the surrounding liver, scan is normal. Normal liver scan plus unsuspected mass on computed tomography (CT) scan indicates focal nodular hyperplasia.
         c. High number shows hot spot; 40% contain enough Kupffer's cells to take up sulfur colloid.

V. Cavernous hemangiomas.
   A. Background.

      1. Most common benign tumor of liver.

        a. Can reach size large enough to cause CHF.

  B. Technique.

      1. Label rbc's (see GI bleeding section).

      2. Place patient under a large-field-of-view camera with a high-resolution low energy parallel-hole collimator.

      3. Perform flow study—one frame per second for 60 seconds.

      4. Image planar views in the appropriate positions for 1,000,000 counts immediately after injection, and at 1 and 2 hours after injection.

      5. Perform SPECT imaging—exact protocol varies with number of heads—for dual-headed camera:

        a. High-resolution, low energy parallel-hole collimator.

        b. 360 degree rotation.

        c. 128 × 128 matrix.

        d. 120 stops; 30 seconds/stop.

  C. Findings.

      1. Hepatic angiogram usually *not* hypervascular. Tumors have increased blood volume, not increased perfusion. Stasis may cause perfusion to appear later than normal parenchyma.

      2. Solitary cold defect—90%; multiple—10%.

      3. Frequently subcapsular; 20% pedunculated.

      4. Blood pool agents such as ^{99m}Tc labeled red cells are useful in diagnosing hemangiomas. Increased blood pool activity seen in face of normal flow.

VI. Abscesses.

  A. Pyogenic.

      1. Background.

        a. Usually occur as complications of abdominal surgery—gastrointestinal or genitourinary.

      2. Findings.

        a. Solitary or multiple cold defects.

          (1) Most commonly in dome of right lobe.

          (2) Usually appear much larger than abscess cavity itself because of inflammation in surrounding liver parenchyma that does not function normally.

        b. If superior dome defect seen without surrounding rim of liver tissue, cannot differentiate from subphrenic abscess.

        c. Should obtain chest x-ray because large pleural effusion, empyema, or lung tumor can produce defect on liver scan.

  B. Amebic.

      1. Background.

            a. Associated with GI amebiasis. Should suspect in endemic areas.

        2. Findings.

            a. Cold defect, almost exclusively posterior right lobe, primarily dome.

            b. Solitary and large.

VII. Cysts.

    A. Echinococcal.

        1. Background.

            a. Rare in United States.

            b. Endemic in underdeveloped countries where cattle and sheep are raised.

            c. Important to consider in differential diagnosis of cold defect, because potential of inadvertently spreading disease by biopsy or laparotomy.

        2. Findings.

            a. Hypovascular.

            b. Cold defect.

            c. Usually solitary, often quite large.

    B. Other cysts.

        1. Polycystic—50% associated with cysts in kidney.

        2. Simple.

        3. All seen as cold defects.

VIII. Traumatic lesions

    A. Lacerations—appear as linear areas of decreased activity.

    B. Hematoma—more circular defect.

    C. Subcapsular hematoma.

        1. Background—occasionally result of liver biopsy in addition to external trauma.

        2. Sensitivity—ultrasound/CT better technique.

        3. Findings—extrinsic mass. Intraparenchymal defect rarely seen.

    D. Hematobilia—cold defect.

Diffuse Liver Disease

  I. Sensitivity—85%. Findings nonspecific. Usually impossible to offer a definitive diagnosis within causes of diffuse liver disease.

 II. Findings.

    A. Inhomogeneity—most common finding.

    B. Hepatomegaly.

    C. Shunting to spleen and bone marrow.

III. Hepatitis.

    A. Background—causes include:

        1. Viral.

        2. Alcoholic.

        3. Other etiologies.

    B. Findings.

        1. Mild-moderate cases.

           a. Moderate inhomogeneity.

           b. Mild-moderate hepatomegaly.

           c. Shunting.

        3. Severe cases.

           a. Hepatic uptake decreased.

           b. More significant hepatomegaly.

           c. Most severe cases—no liver uptake may be seen because of degree of hepatic dysfunction.

        4. Occasional cases associated with small livers without shunting.

        5. Occasionally—small multiple cold focal defects occur. Can be misdiagnosed as mass lesions.

IV. Fatty infiltration.

    A. Background—most commonly due to:

        1. Diabetes.

        2. Alcoholic liver disease.

        3. Total parenteral nutrition.

        4. Obesity.

    B. Findings.

        1. Hepatomegaly—most common.

        2. More severe cases, especially secondary to alcoholism, associated with inhomogeneity and shunting.

        3. May be difficult to differentiate fatty infiltration from acute alcoholic hepatitis in alcoholic liver disease. Shunting makes the latter more likely.

        4. Can be associated with uptake of xenon on ventilation lung studies. This finding can be used for differential diagnosis of inhomogeneity/hepatomegaly.

V. Cirrhosis.

    A. Background—develops as a result of:

        1. Alcoholism—most common cause.

        2. Following hepatitis.

        3. Biliary disease.

    B. Findings.

        1. Early.

           a. Fatty infiltration stage—liver often normal.

           b. Early cirrhosis.

               (1) Atrophy of right lobe with compensatory hypertrophy of left lobe as a result of blood streaming effect in por-

tal vein. High alcohol blood from small intestine (superior mesenteric vein) flows into right lobe. Low alcohol blood (inferior mesenteric vein) streams to left side of portal vein, into the left lobe.

    (2) Shunting—spleen and especially bone marrow. Due to fibrosis developing in liver. Fibrosis increases resistance, causing portal hypertension. Portacaval anastomoses develop. Fibrosis replaces sinusoids. These changes result in decreased hepatic transit of colloid raising blood concentration of sulfur colloid (SC), allowing spleen and bone marrow to extract more SC than usual.

    (3) Splenomegaly. Due to portal hypertension.

  2. Advanced cirrhosis.

    a. Liver shrinks in size.

    b. Cold defect a result of poor function and fibrosis.

    c. Occasional hot defects—regenerating nodules.

    d. Increased separation liver/bone marrow because of ascites.

  3. Final stage of cirrhosis.

    a. Hepatic colloid uptake decreases or becomes zero.

    b. Lung uptake.

    c. Large amount of blood pool activity.

Specific Splenic Diseases

  I. Infarction.

    A. Background.

      1. Most common cause of cold defects in spleen.

    B. Causes.

      1. Subacute bacterial endocarditis.

      2. Massive splenomegaly (myelofibrosis and leukemia).

      3. Hemolytic anemias.

      4. Alcoholism.

      5. Pancreatitis.

    C. Findings.

      1. Cold defect—wedge-shaped, peripheral.

      2. Solitary or multiple.

  II. Hematoma.

    A. Background.

      1. Usually results from trauma or bleeding diathesis.

    B. Sensitivity—excellent.

    C. Specificity—93%.

    D. Findings.

      1. Cold defect—indicates subcapsular or intrapulp bleed.

      2. Linear defect—indicates fracturing of spleen.

3. Splenomegaly.
4. Diffusely diminished sulfur colloid uptake plus splenomegaly. May be seen without focal lesion in diffuse intrasplenic bleeding.

III. Tumors.
  A. Malignant.
    1. Lymphomas—most common tumor; primarily Hodgkin's.
      a. Sensitivity and specificity—low.
      b. Findings.
        (1) Mild-moderate splenomegaly most common finding. Unfortunately, patients may develop reactive splenomegaly *without* actual splenic tumor involvement.
        (2) Cold defects—rare.
    2. Metastases.
      a. Background—rare.
        (1) Breast.
        (2) Lung carcinoma.
        (3) Melanoma.
        (4) Islet cell tumors.
        (5) Gastric or colon carcinomas—occasionally directly invade spleen.
      c. Findings—solitary or multiple cold defects.
    3. Abscesses.
      a. Rare—usually secondary to sepsis (especially endocarditis).
      b. Findings.
        (1) Cold defect—indistinguishable from other causes of cold defects.
    4. Benign tumors.
      a. Causes.
        (1) Hemangioma.
        (2) Fibroma.
        (3) Hamartoma.
    5. Cysts.
      a. Simple cyst—rare.
      b. Echinococcal cysts—occur in hydatid disease.

IV. Functional asplenia.
  A. Background—lack of splenic uptake of sulfur colloid in patients with anatomically intact spleens. These individuals demonstrate Howell-Jolly bodies as one would expect in asplenia.
  B. Causes.
    1. Decreased perfusion.
      a. Sickle cell anemia.
      b. Thalassemia.

2. Diminished RES function.
   a. Tumor replacement.
   b. Thoratrast.
   c. Celiac disease.

Catheter Placement Studies

I. Background.
   A. Used to determine if chemotherapy infusion catheter is in proper position.
   B. Advantage over contrast angiography because contrast studies done with pressure and infusion rate higher than normal. They may not reflect distribution of chemotherapeutic agent at "normal" infusion pump flow rate.
II. Technique.
   A. Technetium macroaggregated albumin (MAA); 1 mCi injected slowly through infusion line. Liver imaging performed.
   B. ^{99m}Tc sulfur colloid then injected IV and imaged.
   C. Computer subtraction of two studies then performed.
III. Findings.
   A. Can determine if tumor being perfused. Can detect if normal parenchyma bypassed.
   B. GI uptake. Presence indicates misplacement of catheter. Gastric or bowel necrosis could occur.
   C. Lung activity. Seen if arteriovenous (AV) shunting present in tumor.

Relationship of Liver-Spleen Scan to CT, Ultrasound, and Liver Function Tests

I. Liver function tests (LFTs).
   A. Patients can have normal LFTs in face of liver metastases.
      1. 36% of patients with metastases had normal alkaline phosphatase levels in one study. Liver-spleen scan detected in 83% of these patients.
      2. Elevated LFTs nonspecific—may be caused by hepatotoxicity from chemotherapeutic agents, etc.
II. CT and ultrasound.
   A. Sensitivity.
      1. CT most sensitive technique for detecting masses.
      2. Radionuclide liver-spleen scan more sensitive than ultrasound.
      3. Sensitivity of radionuclide study for tumor 85% to 90%. SPECT improves sensitivity 5% to 10%.
   B. Ultrasound, CT, radionuclides depend on different parameters for imaging. Occasionally will miss mass on one technique that is obvious on the others.

HEPATOBILIARY IMAGING

Anatomy

(See "Liver-Spleen Scanning.")

Physiology

(See "Liver-Spleen Scanning.")

Radiopharmaceuticals

I. ^{131}I Rose bengal.
   A. Fluoroscein dye tagged with iodine.
   B. Slow hepatic transit time and high radiation dose; limited utility.
II. Iminodiacetic acid.
   A. Analogues of IDA with different end substitutions. Related to lidocaine.
   B. Biliary excretion highest with molecules:
      1. Molecular weight—300 to 1,000.
      2. One portion strongly polar, other lipophilic.
      3. Intramolecular separation of hydrophilic and lipophilic structures.
      4. Stereochemistry with cyclic structure in different planes.
      5. Protein bound.
   C. Clearance.
      1. Removed by hepatocytes through carrier-mediated anionic clearance.
      2. Bilirubin competitive for transport binding sites causing hepatic uptake to fall as bilirubin increases.
   D. HIDA—dimethyl-IDA.
      1. First IDA widely used.
      2. 85% of material excreted by biliary system; 15%, by kidneys.
      3. Useful to bilirubin of 8 mg/dl.
   E. PIPIDA—paraisopropyl IDA.
      1. Higher hepatic extraction because of higher molecular weight and decreased polarity.
      2. Works with bilirubins up to 20 mg/dl.
      3. Duct visualization may be poor, even in normals.
   F. BIDA—parabutyl IDA.
      1. 2% renal excretion.
      2. Useful in patients with bilirubin levels of 10 to 20 mg/dl.
      3. Problems—slow hepatic uptake and excretion.
   G. DISIDA—diisopropyl IDA.
      1. Most commonly used hepatobiliary agent at present.
      2. Higher molecular weight and lipid solubility.

3. Useful to bilirubins of 30 mg/dl. Most rapid hepatic excretion half-time.

Technique

I. Nothing by mouth for 4 to 6 hours. Food stimulates release of cholecystokinin (CCK) causing gallbladder to contract, not allowing IDA to enter.

II. Dose of 3 to 5 mCi ^{99m}Tc IDA injected IV. With elevated bilirubin, dose increased to 10 mCi. Minimum neonatal dose, 1 mCi.

III. Imaging—large-field-of-view camera, parallel-hole low-energy collimator. Liver positioned in right upper portion of field of view. Images 500,000 to 750,000 each every 5 minutes first 30 minutes, every 10 minutes next 30 minutes. Additional images as necessary.

IV. Modifications.
   A. Some centers pretreat with CCK before imaging using 0.2 to 0.4 μg/kg of sincalide (active octapeptide of CCK).
   B. Morphine.
      1. If gallbladder not visualized by 40 minutes, 0.04 mg/kg of morphine given IV causes sphincter of Oddi spasm forcing IDA into gallbladder if cystic duct patent.
      2. Allows rapid differentiation of acute from chronic cholecystitis.
      3. Image for 20 to 50 minutes after morphine injection.
   C. If gallbladder does not visualize by 1 hour (in non-morphine study), additional imaging out to 4 hours is recommended to help differentiate acute from chronic cholecystitis. Also, 24-hour images may be helpful. Prolonged fasting individuals may visualize at 24 hours. Bowel may also visualize in partial duct obstruction or stone being passed.

Normal Scan

I. Early images show liver, cardiac, and vascular activity that fades as hepatic uptake increases. Gallbladder not visualized.

II. Gallbladder and common duct/bowel activity seen by 60 minutes. Gallbladder uptake should precede bowel visualization.

III. Minimal renal activity may occasionally be seen.

IV. As bilirubin increases, less hepatic uptake, more background activity and greater renal excretion seen.

Abnormal Scans

I. Acute cholecystitis.
   A. Background.
      1. Vast majority of cases due to cystic duct obstruction, usually caused by stone.

2. Symptoms.
   a. Nausea.
   b. Vomiting.
   c. Fever.
   d. Right upper quadrant (RUQ) pain.
   e. RUQ tenderness.
2. Sensitivity—acute cholecystitis 95% or greater.
3. Specificity—99% in typical patient.
   a. 10% false-positive rate from chronic cholecystitis. Can be reduced to less than 1% with delayed imaging or morphine.
4. Findings.
   a. Nonvisualization of the gallbladder at 1 hour with normal hepatic uptake and visualization of common duct and bowel.
   b. Nonvisualization of gallbladder at 4 hours (non-morphine study) can occur in:
      (1) Chronic cholecystitis.
      (2) Hyperalimentation.
      (3) Alcoholism.
      (4) Severe intercurrent diseases.
   c. Alternatively, nonvisualization of the gallbladder at 80 to 150 minutes following morphine administration.
   d. May also see nonvisualization of bowel because of choledocholithiasis.
   e. In 3.5%, severe but incomplete cystic duct obstruction caused delayed visualization of gallbladder with acute cholecystitis, indistinguishable from chronic cholecystitis.
5. Secondary signs of acute cholecystitis.
   a. Photopenic defect in gallbladder fossa.
   b. Rim sign.
      (1) Increased uptake in region of gallbladder fossa.
      (2) Caused by either:
         (a) Increased flow.
         (b) Edema bringing about delayed egress of IDA in biliary radicals.
   c. In 7% of cases of acute cholecystitis, small focus of activity seen in region of gallbladder fossa. IDA in cystic duct proximal to obstruction. Comparison of size of gallbladder by ultrasound will differentiate from small fibrotic gallbladder.
II. Gallbladder perforation.
   A. Background.
      1. High mortality without surgical intervention.
      2. May occur without cystic duct obstruction.
      3. Frequently occurs in patients with chronic cholecystitis (which

may be unknown clinically). Primarily elderly patients with severe atherosclerotic disease or immunocompromised patients.

B. Findings.
1. Acute perforation—IDA appearing in gallbladder fossa region—flowing freely into peritoneal cavity.
2. Subacute—pericolic collection.

III. Acute acalculous cholecystitis.
1. Background.
   a. Makes up 5% to 15% of all cases of gallbladder inflammation.
   b. Causes 25% to 45% of postoperative cholecystitis.
   c. Accounts for one third of pediatric cases.
   d. Much poorer prognosis than calculous disease, with half progressing to serious complication.
   e. Predisposing causes include:
      (1) Chemical irritation secondary to hyperconcentrated bile.
      (2) Chemical toxins.
      (3) Bacterial infection.
      (4) Ischemia.
2. Sensitivity of IDA—varies in literature from 45% to 100%; average sensitivity, 80% to 85%.
3. Findings.
   a. Nonvisualization of the gallbladder.
   b. Occasionally—evidence of common duct obstruction.

IV. Chronic cholecystitis.
A. Background.
1. Primarily associated with gallstones.
B. Sensitivity—varies from 10% to 75%, varying with population studied. Patients with more severe, long-standing symptoms have higher percentage of abnormal scans.
C. Findings—two primary patterns.
1. Delayed visualization of the gallbladder due to viscous bile, stones, or fibrosis causing anatomical-functional obstruction. IDA takes course of least resistance, passing through common duct. The more delayed the nonvisualization, the greater the specificity for chronic cholecystitis.
2. Prolonged biliary-to-bowel transit. Perhaps due to ampullitis from inflammation of nearby gallbladder or repeated passage of small stones.
3. Visualization of gallbladder and bowel by 1 hour, but bowel appearing before gallbladder.
   a. Indicates chronic cholecystitis approximately 75% of time.

V. Common duct obstruction.
   A. Background.
      1. May be a result of:
         a. Choledocholithiasis.
         b. Tumor.
         c. Other causes.
      2. Sensitivity—excellent.
      3. Findings—three patterns.
         a. Good hepatic uptake with visualization of gallbladder and common duct, no flow into bowel.
         b. Good hepatic uptake with no visualization of intrahepatic or common bile duct, gallbladder, or bowel. Occurs because intraductal pressures are above secretory pressures of hepatocytes.
         c. Dilated duct. Problem—width of IDA activity in common duct on images is primarily related to amount of radioactivity in duct, less so to actual width.
VI. Biliary enteric bypass patency.
   A. Background—IDA scan can be useful in diagnosing stenosis/obstruction of enteric bypasses postoperatively.
   B. Findings.
      1. Partial bypass obstruction.
         a. Dilated intrahepatic ducts.
         b. Prominent liver activity persisting over 4 hours.
         c. Delayed bowel visualization.
         d. Delayed washout of activity from bypass.
   C. Complete obstruction.
      1. Can appear similar to complete common bile duct obstruction.

Comparison of Cholescintigraphy With Other Radiographic Techniques

  I. Oral cholecystogram.
   A. Based on opacification of gallbladder by iodinated contrast agents.
   B. Dependent on:
      1. Oral ingestion.
      2. Intestinal absorption.
      3. Hepatic conjugation.
   C. Not useful in patients with hyperbilirubinemia or acute symptoms.
 II. Intravenous cholangiography (IVC).
   A. Not useful with even mild elevations of bilirubin.
   B. Many nondiagnostic studies.
   C. Adverse contrast reactions.

III. Ultrasonography.
   A. Depends on indirect signs for diagnosis of acute cholecystitis, i.e., stones plus pain indicate cholecystitis. More direct signs are less common. Unfortunately, approximately 20 million Americans have gallstones.
IV. Comparisons of IDA to ultrasound indicate sensitivity for IDA 98%, ultrasound 81%. Specificity, 90% IDA, 60% ultrasound.
   1. One advantage of ultrasound is that abnormalities in other structures, such as kidney, can be evaluated at the same time.

GASTRIC EMPTYING

Physiology

I. Solids.
   A. Solids must first be reduced to 1.2 mm by grinding action of stomach before can pass through pylorus.
   B. Emptying primarily dependent on antral contraction.
II. Liquids.
   A. Emptying primarily due to gravity.
   B. Therefore solids more sensitive than liquids for detecting abnormal gastric emptying.

Technique

I. Preparation of markers.
   A. In vivo labeled chicken liver.
      1. ^{99m}Tc sulfur colloid injected in wing vein of live chicken. Chicken killed, liver removed and cooked. Fed to patient as solid-phase marker.
      2. Advantage—no elution of tag.
      3. Disadvantage—inconvenient.
   B. In vitro labeled chicken liver.
      1. Fifty grams of paté mixed with 3 mCi of ^{99m}Tc sulfur colloid.
      2. Incubated 10 minutes, then placed in hot pan and stir-fried 10 to 15 minutes.
      3. Advantages—convenience, little elution of tag.
      4. Disadvantage—aerosolization of tag when cooked.
   C. Liquid marker.
      1. ^{111}In mixed in orange juice.
II. Administration of meal.
   A. Patient must have had nothing by mouth for 8 hours.
   B. Patient consumes meal as quickly as possible. We use standard 300-g meal. Rate of emptying varies with caloric content, so must standardize.

III. Imaging.
   A. At meal conclusion and 10- or 20-minute intervals.
   B. Subject is imaged in upright position using large-field-of-view camera and medium energy colimator. Anterior and posterior images obtained using separate 140- and 247-keV photopeaks.
   C. External ^{99m}Tc point source taped to patient's abdomen to allow accurate horizontal and vertical repositioning for each set of images.
   D. Data stored on magnetic disk of computer.
IV. Imaging processing.
   A. Region of interest over stomach selected from composite of anterior and posterior technetium images.
   B. Data corrected for radionuclide cross-talk. This is downscatter of 173- and 247-keV photons of indium 111 into 140-keV window of pertechnetate. Determined by phantom studies, what percentage of counts in technetium window occur from set dose of ^{111}In.
   C. Correction made for technetium decay (6-hour half-life).
   D. Correction for depth. Gastric fundus more posterior than antrum. With anterior imaging, counts will increase as label moves more distally. Corrected with geometric mean—square root of anterior times posterior counts.
   E. Emptying curve (percent retention vs. time).
      1. T$\frac{1}{2}$ determined.

Normal Study

I. Curve shapes.
   A. Solids—linear.
   B. Liquids—monoexponential.
II. Meal size: the larger the meal size, the slower the gastric emptying.
III. Caloric content: the greater the caloric content, the slower the gastric emptying.
IV. For these reasons, gastric emptying meals must be standardized.
V. Males.
   A. No variation with age.
VI. Females.
   A. Premenopausal—solids and liquids empty more slowly than in men because of intestinal smooth-muscle relaxation caused by estradiol and progesterone.
   B. Postmenopausal—same rate as men.

Abnormal Study

I. Mechanical obstruction.

A. Solids—always delayed.

B. Liquids—may empty normally.

II. Altered function (e.g., diabetic gastroparesis.)

A. Solids—delayed.

B. Liquids—delayed.

III. Causes of delayed gastric emptying.

A. Diabetes mellitus.

B. Surgery (postsurgical period).

C. Drugs.

D. Gastric outlet obstruction.

E. Scleroderma.

F. Chronic ideopathic intestinal pseudo-obstruction (CIIP).

G. Ideopathic gastroparesis.

H. Amyloidosis.

I. Anorexia nervosa.

IV. Dumping syndrome.

A. Rapid solid and liquid emptying.

MECKEL'S DIVERTICULUM SCANNING

Anatomy

I. Meckel's diverticulum most common congenital anomaly of GI tract; occurs in 2% of population.

II. Remnant of omphalomesenteric or vitelline duct. This duct arises from fetal yolk sac and connects umbilicus with fetal intestine.

III. Meckel's diverticulum found on antimesenteric side of terminal ileum within 45 to 90 cm of ileocecal valve.

IV. Measures 1 to 12 cm long (average, 6 cm). Sometimes connected by fibrous band to anterior abdominal wall at umbilicus.

V. Twenty-five percent contain ectopic mucosa; these have propensity to bleed. Pancreatic, duodenal, colonic mucosa also found.

Physiology

I. Ectopic gastric mucosa concentrates ^{99m}Tc just as normal gastric mucosa does. Mucus secretory cells, not parietal and chief cells, concentrate pertechnetate.

II. Background.

A. Most with Meckel's asymptomatic.

B. Four percent become symptomatic, causing bleeding, intussusception, volvulus, or diverticulitis.

C. Majority symptomatic by 2 years of age.

D. Bleeding painless in distinction to intussusception. Bleeding caused by hydrochloric acid and pepsin secreted by ectopic gastric mucosa ulcerating adjacent mucosa.

III. Rule of 2's for Meckel's diverticulum.
   A. Occur in 2% of population.
   B. Occur within 2 feet of the ileocecal valve.
   C. Average 2 inches in length.
   D. Usually symptomatic by age 2.

Technique

   I. Nothing by mouth for preceding 6 to 12 hours.
   II. ^{99m}Tc pertechnetate 200 µCi/kg or 10 mCi in adults.
   III. Angiogram—5-second anterior abdominal images for 60 seconds. Screening for vascular lesions that may cause bleeding. Meckel's diverticula, unless actively bleeding at time of study, are negative on this phase of study.
   IV. Delayed imaging—large-field-of-view camera (for adults) used with stomach in left upper portion of field (bladder, lower field of view). Imaged every 5 minutes for minimum of 1 hour. Additional delayed anterior, oblique, lateral views obtained as necessary. Since Meckel's diverticula can lie on bladder, a postvoid film should also be obtained.
   V. Modifications.
   A. Patient may be positioned on left side at 45- to 90-degree tilt to decrease emptying of pertechnetate from stomach into bowel.
   B. Nasogastric (NG) tube placed. Again, to decrease peristalsis of normally secreted pertechnetate into GI tract.
   C. Pharmacologic intervention.
      1. Glucagon—50 µg to 1 mg given. Promotes pooling and prevents downstream wash of pertechnetate.
      2. Pentagastrin—6 µg/kg. Increases uptake of pertechnetate by 30% to 60%. Since glucagon causes mild decrease of pertechnetate uptake, glucagon and pentagastrin are often combined.
      3. Cimetidine—300 mg four times a day 1 to 2 days before performing scan. Histamine antagonist. Blocks secretion pertechnetate from gastric mucosa improving lesion/background ratio.
      4. Ranitidine.
         a. May have fewer side effects than cimetidine.
         b. Infuse 1 mg/kg (maximum of 50 mg) over 20 minutes.
         c. Begin imaging 1 hour later.

Normal Study

   I. Increased gastric uptake is seen over first 10 to 20 minutes. With time, pertechnetate may leave stomach and undergo peristalsis distally. Usually appears linear, but occasionally focal.
   II. Renal activity seen in early part of examination. Common cause of false-positve findings. Especially focal and prominent with extrarenal pelvis. Oblique, lateral, and posterior views show activity far poste-

rior, indicating GU activity rather than Meckel's diverticulum. Occasionally, ureter visualizes focally as it passes over pelvic brim. This activity will diminish as study progresses.

III. Bladder activity normally seen. Identified by location and increasing size as study progresses.

Abnormal Study

I. Focally increased activity not associated with normal structures.

II. Timing.

    A. Activity in Meckel's diverticula will first appear at same time pertechnetate appears in normal gastric mucosa of stomach (usually 5 to 20 minutes following injection). Activity increases with time paralleling stomach.

III. Location.

    A. Usually right lower quadrant. May be close to bladder. Rarely located in other areas of abdomen.

IV. Size.

    A. Small and focal. Although Meckel's diverticulum is a tube, ectopic gastric mucosa forms only a small patch of tissue within Meckel's diverticulum. Therefore tubular activity more likely to represent normal bowel activity or ectopic gastric mucosa in intestinal duplication.

V. Intensity.

    A. Activity will increase with time or remain the same. Renal activity fades. Occasionally, downstream wash of pertechnetate will cause Meckel's diverticula to decrease with time.

VI. Lack of peristalsis.

    A. Meckel's diverticulum activity remains in the same location. Normal bowel activity moves due to peristalsis.

VII. Change of position.

    A. Meckel's diverticulum—like bowel, will move with change in patient's position. Retroperitoneal renal activity will not move.

    B. Problem—some Meckel's diverticula attached to anterior abdominal wall by fibrous cord. These will not move.

VIII. Utility of study.

    A. Sensitivity—85%+.

    B. Specificity—95%.

    C. False-negative results due to:

        1. Small size.

        2. Absence gastric mucosa.

        3. Autonecrosis of gastric mucosa.

        4. Rapid downstream wash of pertechnetate.

        5. Obscured by activity in normal structures.

D. False-positives caused by:
  1. Normal activity.
     a. GI tract.
     b. Bladder.
     c. Renal.
  2. Ectopic gastric mucosa.
     a. Intestinal duplication.
     b. Gastrogenic cysts.
  3. Increased blood pool resulting from inflammation.
     a. Intussusception.
     b. Appendicitis.
  3. Hypervascularity.
     a. Tumor.
     b. Arteriovenous malformation.

BARRETT'S ESOPHAGUS

I. Background.
  A. Replacement of normal stratified squamous epithelium of distal esophagus by columnar epithelium similar to gastric mucosa.
  B. Associated with esophagitis and ulceration.
  C. Uptake of pertechnetate occurs in abnormal esophageal mucosa.
  D. Technique—modified Meckel's diverticulum scan.
     1. Have patient drink water to prevent swallowed salivary gland secretions from causing false-positive.
II. Modified Meckel's diverticulum scan occasionally used to determine if patient who has undergone gastrectomy had incomplete antrectomy (retained gastric antrum), which can cause elevated gastric acid level and ulceration.

ESOPHAGEAL MOTILITY STUDIES

Physiology

I. Decreased esophageal motility seen with:
  A. Achalasia.
  B. Scleroderma.
  C. Diffuse esophageal spasm.

Technique

I. Patient has nothing by mouth overnight.
II. Patient ingests through a straw 150 μCi of ^{99m}Tc sulfur colloid diluted in 15 ml H_2O in a single swallow. Subject continues to dry-swallow at 15-second intervals for 10 minutes. Counts over esophagus stored in computer.

III. Count rate within area used to calculate rate of esophageal transit using formula:

$$ET = \frac{E\ max - EC}{E\ max \times 100}$$

where ET indicates percent of esophageal transit at time T; E max = maximum count rate in esophagus; and EC = esophageal count at time T.

Normal Studies

I. Esophageal activity decreases very rapidly; 5 to 10 seconds after first swallow, activity not visible on camera, although low count rates detectable by computer. After eight swallows, transit rates greater than 90% in normals.

Abnormal Study

I. Transit rate 5% to 40% after eight swallows—note diffuse esophageal spasm has significantly reduced rate first half of study, normal after 20 swallows.
II. Sensitivity.
   A. Much more sensitive than manometry. Picks up two thirds of dysphagic patients with normal manometry because pressure waves recorded by manometry do not always correlate with force applied in aboral direction to solid bolus.

ESOPHAGEAL REFLUX STUDIES

Background

I. Heartburn/regurgitation—one of the most common diseases. One third of individuals symptomatic at least once a month.

Technique

I. Patient takes orally 300 µCi of ^{99m}Tc sulfur colloid in 300 ml of acidified orange juice.
II. Ten to 15 minutes later, patient imaged in upright position. If activity in esophagus seen, attempt made to clear it with water.
III. After initial image, abdominal binder used to sequentially increase lower esophageal sphincter pressure in 5 mm Hg steps up to 100. Images recorded on computer for 30 seconds at each pressure station.
IV. Reflux calculated at each pressure step using formula:

$$R = (ET - EB)/G_0 \times 100$$

where R indicates percent gastroesophageal reflux; ET = esophageal count at time T; EB = esophageal background counts; and G_0 gastric counts at beginning of study.

V. Sensitivity—reflux detected in 90% of symptomatic patients. Much more sensitive than fluoroscopy and endoscopy (40% sensitivity) and lower esophageal sphincter pressure measurement. Similar in sensitivity to acid reflux test.

Pediatric Patients

I. Background.
   A. Reflux in infants different entity than in adults. Occurs in healthy infants. Frequency and extent of reflux separates significant from insignificant reflux.
   B. Sequelae significant. Reflux in children causes:
      1. Failure to thrive.
      2. Aspiration pneumonia.
      3. Esophagitis.
      4. Stricture.
II. Technique.
   A. Similar to adult technique. Material may be instilled via intubation or mixed with formula.
III. Gastric emptying study combined with esophageal examination since delayed gastric emptying has been linked to reflux.

GASTROINTESTINAL TRACT BLEEDING

Anatomy and Physiology

I. Upper GI tract bleeding.
   A. Proximal to ligament of Treitz.
   B. Common causes.
      1. Gastric ulcers.
      2. Duodenal ulcers.
      3. Gastritis.
      4. Varices.
II. Lower GI tract bleeding.
   A. Distal to ligament of Treitz.
   B. Causes.
      1. Diverticula.
      2. Angiodysplasia.
      3. Inflammatory bowel disease.
      4. Neoplasms.
III. Special groups of patients.
   A. Pediatric.
      1. Upper GI—same as adults.
      2. Lower GI.
         a. Meckel's diverticulum.

      b. Intussusception.

      c. Juvenile polyps.

  B. Renal transplant.

    1. Upper GI—peptic ulcer disease.

    2. Lower GI—cecal ulceration.

  C. Tumor patients.

    1. Upper GI and lower GI—usual causes most common. Hemorrhage secondary to solid tumor in 17% to 55%.

  D. Severely stressed patients.

    1. Upper GI—"stress ulcers."

  E. Drug-associated hemorrhage.

    1. Upper GI—0.3%—heparin, warfarin, corticosteroids, ethacrynic acid, aspirin.

^{99m}Tc Sulfur Colloid Studies

  I. Theory.

    A. Small amount of injected sulfur colloid extravasates with each circulation until sulfur colloid cleared by RES. Normal clearance results in high target-to-background ratio.

 II. Technique.

    A. Ten to 15 mCi of sulfur colloid injected IV. High doses used to increase photon flux, because only small amount of tag extravasated.

    B. Angiogram performed every 5 seconds for 60 seconds. May detect bleeding site on flow study.

    C. Static images. Small portion of lower edge of liver is placed in upper field of view. Images obtained every 1 to 2 minutes for 30 minutes then at 45 minutes and 1 hour for 500,000 to 1,000,000 counts each. Delayed imaging done to allow sulfur colloid that may have extravasated in hepatic or splenic flexures and would be obscured by normal liver and spleen activity to move into view.

    D. Oblique and lateral views of upper part of abdomen should be performed to look for higher bleeding sites if lower images negative.

III. Normal study.

    A. Flow study.

      1. No evidence of focally increased activity.

    B. Static images.

      1. Blood pool that quickly fades.

      2. Mild marrow uptake seen.

      3. Edges of iliacs may be misinterpreted as a hemorrhage if patient in oblique position.

      4. Bladder occasionally seen, depending on adequacy of tag.

      5. In males, linear activity representing blood pool in penis is frequently seen.

IV. Abnormal.
    A. Flow study.
        1. Focal area of increased activity.
    B. Statics
        1. Focal area of increased activity that becomes more intense on first few images. Will undergo peristalsis and move distally on subsequent images. Pattern of movement helpful in differentiating small bowel from colon.
    V. Sensitivity—in dog studies, 0.05 to .1 ml/minute bleeds detected. Sulfur colloid scan twice as sensitive for detecting GI bleeding in patients as contrast angiogram.
    A. Upper GI bleeding likely to be missed because of normal liver and spleen activity.
    B. Very low rectal hemorrhages may be missed. Cause unknown; may be due to attenuation from pelvic structures. Stools passed during examination should be imaged to detect these hemorrhages.

^{99m}Tc-Labeled Red Blood Cells

I. Background.
    A. Extravasated cells show up as focal hot spot after sufficient number accumulate. With red blood cells labeled, background activity higher than sulfur colloid.
    B. Longer imaging times required to detect slow bleeding rate.
    C. Tag adequate for 24 hours, allowing intermittent bleeds to be reimaged without reinjection.
II. Technique.
    A. Red blood cells can be labeled, using in vivo, modified in vitro, or in vitro techniques (see Chapter 8).
        1. Because in vitro technique has best labeling efficiency (98%), it is preferred technique; 20 to 30 mCi used for labeling.
    B. Flow study performed as in sulfur colloid study.
    C. Nasogastric suction should be performed with in vivo tagging. 50% of normals will show GI activity over 24 hours if suction not used.
    D. Large-field-of-view camera over anterior abdomen. Immediate blood pool image for 500-K counts, then 1 to 5 minutes for 90 to 120 minutes. Re-image as necessary if patient is thought to have hemorrhage again up to 24 hours following labeling.
III. Normal scan.
    A. Heart and great vessels prominent. Bladder may be seen, especially with in vivo labeling. Bowel activity may be seen on later images. Penile activity frequently seen as in sulfur colloid scan.
IV. Abnormal findings.

A. Flow study.
   1. Focus of increased activity.
B. Static images.
   1. Focal area of activity peristalses with time.
   2. If doesn't move, likely because of vascular activity.
   3. May require imaging up to 4 hours to become positive with slow hemorrhages.
V. Sensitivity—91%; specificity—95%.
   A. In dog study, were able to detect bleeding rates similar to sulfur colloid, although longer imaging times out to 1 hour required. In humans, it has been estimated scan can image bleeds of 500 ml/24 hours or less.
VI. If focus of activity seen when patient is re-imaged for suspected repeat bleeding episode, bleeding site could be more proximal. Occasionally activity undergoes peristalsis in both directions; therefore, one cannot be sure of origin of bleeding site.

Comparison of Sulfur Colloid and Labeled Cells

I. Sensitivity for hemorrhages of 0.05 to .1 ml/minute possible with both. Red blood cells require approximately 3 ml of blood to accumulate, so may take 60 minutes or longer.
II. Red blood cells superior in intermittent bleeding episodes. Can be re-imaged without reinjection. Note that reinjection of second dose of sulfur colloid can be performed, however.
III. Red blood cells superior in upper GI hemorrhages.
IV. Red blood cells have greater potential for false-positive findings because of normal vascular structures and free pertechnetate.
V. Large multiinstitutional study in which both tests were performed on patients found sensitivity of sulfur colloid scan only 12% compared to 93% with labeled red blood cells.

GALLIUM IMAGING
Mechanism of Action

I. Injected intravenously, binds primarily to transferrin, beta-globulin responsible for transporting iron. Patients with hemochromatosis and saturated transferrin iron-binding sites show decreased soft tissue localization of gallium and increased renal excretion of the unbound gallium.
II. Excretion is 15% to 25% of gallium 67 by kidneys in first 24 hours; after 24 hours colon becomes major route of excretion.
III. Gallium distributed throughout plasma and body tissues. Biologic half-life—25 days.

IV. Normal tissues that concentrate gallium have large concentration of lactoferrin—protein with high affinity for gallium. This accounts for uptake seen in lacrimal and salivary glands, nasopharynx, bone marrow, and spleen.

V. Liver metabolizes both lactoferrin and transferrin, explaining its large accumulation.

VI. Intracellular gallium associated with lysosomes and rough-surfaced endoplasmic reticulum.

VII. In inflammatory lesions, gallium is bound to lactoferrin in neutrophils. In addition, gallium can localize in abscesses in aneutropenic animals. Interestingly, bacteria themselves can take up gallium directly.

VIII. Tumors—gallium-transferrin complex binds to specific transferrin receptor on cell surface. Complex is then taken up intact. Gallium initially deposited in the lysomes. This mechanism similar to that proposed for iron uptake in reticulocytes.

Technique

I. Use large-field-of-view camera with triple-window capacity.

II. For inflammatory imaging, 3 to 6 mCi; 10 mCi for tumor imaging in some cases.

III. Need for bowel preparation debatable. Several studies failed to show any real effectiveness in eliminating colonic activity with laxatives or enemas.

IV. Scanning normally done at 24 to 48 hours. Six-hour images useful in infection. Delayed imaging up to 120 hours possible. In neoplastic disease, single 48- or 72-hour images sufficient.

V. Views obtained depend on circumstances for scan. In whole-body evaluation, anterior and posterior views of head, neck, chest, and abdomen with anterior views of extremities. Additional oblique and lateral views as necessary.

Normal Scan

I. Prominent soft-tissue activity present on 6- and 24-hour scans because of slow blood clearance.

II. Renal activity common at 24 hours; may be seen faintly at 48 hours. Represents normal excretion.

III. Bowel activity should decrease and change location on delayed images. Occasionally, it is so intense that it mimics diffuse bowel localization such as pseudomembranous colitis or diffuse peritonitis. Can administer sulfur colloid orally to determine if activity intraluminal.

IV. Areas with high lactoferrin content, lacrimal glands, salivary glands, visualize.

V. Breast, especially in pregnancy, menarche, or patients taking birth control pills, also visualize.
VI. Liver and splenic activity usually seen.
VII. Lung activity occasionally seen on 6- and 24-hour images, fading on delayed views. Prominent pulmonary uptake may be seen on scans performed after lymphangiography.
VIII. Uptake in sternum may mimic mediastinal tumor.
IX. Normally, uptake in the thymus.
X. Epiphyseal uptake common.
XI. Surgical wounds usually positive for 1 week.

Abnormal Studies

I. Inflammatory disease.
  A. Sensitivity—90%.
  B. Most common causes for false-negative study:
    1. Small size abscess.
    2. Leukopenia.
    3. Obscured by organs containing normal uptake.
    4. Not imaging the area involved.
    5. Gallium uptake in liver abscess can be same as surrounding liver; therefore, sulfur colloid scan should also be performed.
  C. Amebic abscesses.
    1. Findings.
      a. "Rim sign"—peripheral shell of activity with cold center. Sign not pathognomonic. Can be seen in large bacterial abscesses and necrotic tumors.
      b. Cause—surrounding hyperemia with avascular center into which gallium cannot penetrate.
  D. Perinephric abscesses/pyelonephritis.
    1. Uptake past normal 24 to 48 hours.
    2. False-positive causes (i.e., non-infectious).
      a. Acute tubular necrosis.
      b. Vasculitis.
      c. Interstitial nephritis.
      d. Amyloidosis.
      e. Obstruction.
      f. Tumor.
      g. Renal transplants.
        (1) Can have positive uptake as a result of:
          (a) Acute tubular necrosis.
          (b) Rejection.
  E. Osteomyelitis and septic arthritis.
    1. Can be helpful if bone scan questionable.

F. Acquired immunodeficiency syndrome (AIDS).
  1. Background.
    a. Caused by a human T-cell lymphotrophic retrovirus.
    b. Retrovirus capable of replicating in a limited number of cell types.
      (1) Lymphocytes.
      (2) Macrophages.
      (3) CNS tissue.
    c. High-risk individuals for AIDS:
      (1) Homosexuals.
      (2) IV drug abusers.
      (3) Recipients of multiple blood transfusions.
      (4) Infants of mothers with AIDS.
  2. *Pneumocystis carinii* pulmonary infections (PCP).
    a. Background.
      (1) In as many as two thirds of cases, *Pneumocystis carinii* infections are initial presentation of AIDS.
      (2) One of main causes of death in AIDS patients.
      (3) Presents with:
        (a) Fever.
        (b) Mild, nonproductive cough.
        (c) Dyspnea.
        (d) Tachypnea.
    b. Role of Gallium 67.
      (1) ^{67}Ga is abnormal in 85% to 95% of cases.
      (2) A normal chest x-ray examination and ^{67}Ga scan make PCP very unlikely.
      (3) In 10% to 20% or more of PCP cases, ^{67}Ga scan is abnormal in the face of a normal chest x-ray examination.
      (4) Specificity varies with criteria used to interpret scan (see below).
      (5) Findings:
        (a) Diffuse bilateral pulmonary uptake.
        (b) Intensity greater than liver—specificity of 90%.
        (c) Lesser degrees of intensity—specificity as low as 50% (sensitivity rises, however).
          (i) Note that occasional cases of fatal PCP have been associated with low grades of ^{67}Ga uptake.
          (ii) Recurrences after treatment may have lesser degrees of uptake.
        (d) Specificity also increases if:

(i) Heterogenous uptake.

(ii) Concurrent chest x-ray examination normal.

(e) Other diseases that can result in diffuse lung uptake:

(i) Cytomegalic virus.

(ii) Smoker's pneumonitis.

(iii) Lymphocytic interstitial pneumonitis.

(iv) Post-drug treatment.

(v) Other ^{67}Ga avid disorders.

3. Other pulmonary infections.

a. *Mycobacterium avium-intracellulare.*

(1) Causes widespread disease in 25% to 50% of AIDS patients.

(2) Uptake in lobar or asymmetric pattern.

(3) Hilar nodes and extra-hilar involvement.

(i) Extra-hilar involvement makes atypical infection more likely than TB.

(ii) Other granulomatous disease (e.g., histoplasmosis) will appear similar.

b. Bacterial infection.

(1) Pattern—lobar involvement without nodal uptake.

c. Cytomegalovirus.

(1) Multiple organ uptake in addition to lungs.

(2) Lung + eye (retinitis) + adrenal (adrenalitis) + renal + colonic.

d. Lymphocytic interstitial pneumonitis—can mimic pulmonary infection.

(1) Diffuse lung uptake + increased parotid uptake.

e. Kaposi's sarcoma—can mimic infection on chest x-ray examination.

(1) Does not cause ^{67}Ga uptake.

4. CNS

a. ^{67}Ga not very useful for detecting CNS infections.

5. GI

a. ^{67}Ga usually negative in Kaposi's sarcoma.

II. Neoplasia.

A. Main interest has been diagnosis and staging lymphomas, especially Hodgkin's disease.

1. Seventy-five percent of sites involved with tumor identified by scan.

2. Less than 6% false-positive rate.

3. Twenty-six percent of asymptomatic patients following therapy had lesions discovered with gallium.

4. Most accurate for nodular sclerosing—89%; least accurate—lymphocyte predominant—75%.
5. Best—thorax—90%. Worst—abdomen—48%.
6. Spleen—only 37% had positive scan with splenic involvement.

B. Lung carcinoma.
   1. Used for staging lung carcinoma. Use is controversial.
   2. Ninety percent of primary lung tumors can be diagnosed. Those missed usually less than 2 cm.
   3. Sensitivity for adenocarcinomas may be less than that of other histologic types.
   4. Results using gallium for staging (detection of hilar and/or mediastinal metastases) have varied. Sensitivities of 30% to 100% and specificities of 63% to 93%.
   5. Whole-body gallium scintigraphy may be helpful in identifying clinically occult metastases of lung carcinoma outside the thorax.

C. Primary hepatoma.
   1. High incidence of alcoholic cirrhosis in the United States and its association with hepatoma creates suspicion of hepatoma far more often than it occurs. Pseudotumors and/or regenerating nodules make diagnosing or excluding hepatoma on sulfur colloid liver scan, CT, and ultrasonography difficult.
   2. In face of cold lesion on ^{99m}Tc sulfur colloid, uptake of ^{67}Ga points toward hepatoma (or inflammation).
   3. Can see gallium uptake in regenerating nodules and metastases. However, degree of uptake usually less than with hepatoma.
   4. Sensitivity—90% (50% of metastases show positive gallium 67 as well).

D. Malignant melanoma.
   1. With SPECT imaging, overall sensitivity of 82% and specificity of 99%. With planar imaging, sensitivity of 54% to 79%. False-positive diagnoses are rare.
   2. Bone, brain, and lung metastases usually detected. Sensitivity falls as lesion size shrinks below 2 cm.
   3. In patients presenting with clinically localized primary tumors, detection of bone, brain, or liver metastases unusual.

E. Gastrointestinal tract tumors.
   1. Normal GI uptake in addition to liver and spleen uptake make imaging tumors of GI tract difficult.
   2. Low sensitivity for gastric and colonic carcinoma.
   3. Relatively insensitive for primary esophageal carcinoma (<50%). Sensitivity greatest when extramural extension has occurred.

   F. Genitourinary tumors.
1. Low sensitivity in kidney, bladder, and prostate carcinoma.
2. Testicular carcinoma—especially seminoma—^{67}Ga may be useful.
3. Not useful in differential diagnosis. May be helpful in identifying metastases.

   G. Head and neck tumors.
1. Variable opinions on effectiveness. Positive scans found in 48% to 84% of squamous cell carcinomas and adenocarcinomas of the head and neck. Lesions less than 1.5 cm not imaged.
2. False-positive diagnoses may occur because of physiologic uptake in nasopharynx and salivary glands. Parotid uptake following radiation due to radiation sialadenitis may be misdiagnosed as tumor infiltration.

   H. Miscellaneous tumors.
1. Not helpful in evaluation of most gynecologic tumors, breast cancer, thyroid cancer, and neuroblastoma.

SUGGESTED READINGS

Alavi A: Detection of gastrointestinal bleeding with ^{99m}Tc-sulfur colloid. *Semin Nucl Med* 1982; 12:126-138.

Alavi A, Dann RW, Baum S, et al: Scintigraphic detection of acute gastrointestinal bleeding. *Radiology* 1977; 124:753-756.

Beckerman C, Bitran J: Gallium-67 scanning in clinical evaluation of human immunodeficiency virus infection: Indications and limitations. *Semin Nucl Med* 1988; 18:273-286.

Beckerman C, Hoffer PB, Bitran JD: The role of gallium-67 in the clinical evaluation of cancer. *Semin Nucl Med* 1985; 15:72-103.

Biello DR, Levitt RG, Melson GI: The roles of gallium-67 scintigraphy, ultrasonography, and computed tomography in the detection of abdominal abscesses. *Semin Nucl Med* 1979; 9:58-65.

Brendel AJ, Leccia F, Drouillard J, et al: Single photon emission computed tomography (SPECT), planar scintigraphy, and transmission computed tomography: A comparison of accuracy in diagnosing focal hepatic disease. *Radiology* 1984; 153:527-532.

Carrasquillo JA, Rogers JV, Schuman WP, et al: Single-photon emission computed tomography of the normal liver. *Am J Radiol* 1983; 141:937-941.

Choy D, Shi EC, McLean RG: Cholescintigraphy in acute cholecystitis: Use of intravenous morphine. *Radiology* 1984; 151:203-207.

Christian PE, Datz FL, Sorenson JA, et al: Technical factors in gastric emptying studies. *J Nucl Med* 1983; 24:264-268.

Datz FL: Role of radionuclide studies in esophageal disease. *J Nucl Med* 1984; 25:1040-1045.

Datz FL: Gastrointestinal imaging. In Taylor AT, Datz FL (eds): *Clinical practice of nuclear medicine*. New York, Churchill-Livingstone, 1991, pp 317-360.

Datz FL, Christian PE, Hutson WR, et al: Physiological and pharmacological interventions in radionuclide imaging of the tubular gastrointestinal tract. *Semin Nucl Med* 1991; 21:140-152.

Datz FL, Christian PE, Moore J: Gender-related differences in gastric emptying. *J Nucl Med* 1987; 28:1204-1207.

Fisher RS, Malmud LS, Roberts GS, et al: Gastroesophageal (GE) scintiscanning to detect and quantitate GE reflux. *Gastroenterology* 1976; 70:302-398.

Freitas FE, Fing-Bennett DM, Thrall JH, et al: Efficacy of hepatobiliary imaging in acute abdominal pain: Concise communication. *J Nucl Med* 1980; 21:919-924.

Ganz WI, Serafini AN: Diagnostic role of nuclear medicine in acquired immunodeficiency syndrome. *J Nucl Med* 1989; 30:1935-1945.

Habibian MR, Staab EV, Matthews HA: Gallium citrate Ga-67 scans in febrile patients. *JAMA* 1975; 233:1073-1076.

Harbert JC: Efficacy of liver scanning in malignant diseases. *Semin Nucl Med* 1984; 14:287-295.

Hoffer PB: Mechanisms of localization. In Hoffer PB, Beckerman C, Henkin RE (eds): *Gallium-67 Imaging*. New York, John Wiley & Sons, 1978, pp 3-8.

Kalff V, Satterlee W, Harkness BA, et al: Liver-spleen studies with the rotating gamma camera. I. Utility of the rotating display. *Radiology* 1984; 153:533-536.

Keyes JW, Singer D, Satterlee W, et al: Liver-spleen studies with the rotating gamma camera. II. Utility of tomography. *Radiology* 1984; 153:537-541.

Kim EF, Hayne TP: Role of nuclear medicine in chemotherapy of malignant lesions. *Semin Nucl Med* 1984; 15:12-20.

Loberg M, Cooper M, Harvey E, et al: Development of a new radiopharmaceutical based on N-substitution of iminodiacetic acid. *J Nucl Med* 1976; 17:633-638.

Malmud LS, Fisher RS, Knight LC, et al: Scintigraphic evaluation of gastric emptying. *Semin Nucl Med* 1982; 12:116-125.

McClees EC, Gedgaudes-McClees RK: Screening for diffuse and focal liver disease: The case for hepatic scintigraphy. *J Clin Ultrasound* 1984; 12:75-81.

McNeil BJ, Sanders R, Alderson PO, et al: A prospective study of computed tomography, ultrasound, and gallium imaging in patients with fever. *Radiology* 1981; 139:647-653.

Miller RF: Nuclear medicine and AIDS. *Eur J Nucl Med* 1990; 16:103-118.

Patton DD: Current status of liver scintigraphy for space-occupying disease. In Freeman LM, Weissman HS (eds): *Nuclear medicine annual 1982*. New York, Raven. pp 35-79.

Pettigrew RI, Witztum KF, Perkins GC, et al: Single photon emission computed tomograms of the liver: Normal vascular intrahepatic structures. *Radiology* 1984; 150:219-223.

Pinsky S, Johnson PM: Radiocolloid imaging of the liver. In Freeman LM (ed): *Freeman and Johnson's clinical radionuclide imaging*, ed 3. New York, Grune & Stratton, 1984, pp 835-878.

Rabinowitz SA, McKusick KA, Strauss HW: ^{99m}Tc red blood cell scintigraphy in evaluating focal liver lesions. *Am J Radiol* 1984; 143:63-68.

Shuman WP, Gibbs R, Rudd TG, et al: PIPIDA scintigraphy for cholecystitis: False positive in alcoholism and total parenteral nutrition. *AJR* 1982; 138:1.

Siemsen JK, Siegfried GF, Waxman AD: The use of Ga-67 in pulmonary disorders. *Semin Nucl Med* 1978; 3:235-249.

Spencer RF, Johnson PM: The spleen. In Freeman LM (ed): *Freeman and Johnson's clinical radionuclide imaging,* ed 3. New York, Grune & Stratton, 1984, pp 1241-1274.

Taylor AT, Datz FL: Gallium imaging in neoplastic and inflammatory disease. In Taylor AT, Datz FL (eds): *Clinical practice of nuclear medicine.* New York, Churchill-Livingstone, 1991, pp. 361-378.

Thorne DA, Datz FL, Remley K, et al: Bleeding rates necessary for detecting acute gastrointestinal bleeding with technetium-99m-labeled red blood cells in an experimental mode. *J Nucl Med* 1987; 28:514-520.

Tolin R, Malmud LS, Reilley J, et al: Esophageal scintigraphy to quantitate the rate of esophageal emptying. *Gastroenterology* 1979; 76:1402-1408.

Tsan MF: Mechanism of gallium-67 accumulation in inflammatory lesions. *J Nucl Med* 1985; 26:88-92.

Waxman AD: Scintigraphic evaluation of diffuse hepatic disease. *Semin Nucl Med* 1982; 12:75-85.

Weissman HS, Badia J, Sugarman LA, et al: Spectrum of 99m-Tc-IDA cholescintigraphic patterns in acute cholecystitis. *Radiology* 1981; 138:167-175.

Weissman HS, Berkowitz D, Fox M, et al: The role of technetium-99m-iminodiacetic acid (IDA) cholescintigraphy in acute acalculous cholecystitis. *Radiology* 1983; 146:177-180.

Weissman HS, Frank MS, Bernstein LH, et al: Rapid and accurate diagnosis of acute cholecystitis with ^{99m}Tc-HIDA cholescintigraphy. *AJR* 1979; 132:523-528.

Weissman HS, Freeman LM: Biliary tract. In Freeman LM (ed): *Freeman and Johnson's clinical radionuclide imaging,* ed 3. New York, Grune & Stratton, 1984, pp 879-1049.

Weissman HS, Gliedman ML, Wilk PJ, et al: Evaluation of the postoperative patient with ^{99m}Tc-IDA cholescintigraphy. *Semin Nucl Med* 1982; 12:27-52.

Weissman HS, Sugarman LA, Frank MS, et al: Serendipity in technetium-99m dimethyl iminodiacetic acid cholescintigraphy. *Radiology* 1980; 135:449-454.

Welch TJ, Sheedy PF, Stephens DH, et al: Focal nodular hyperplasia and hepatic adenoma: Comparison of angiography, CT, US, and scintigraphy. *Radiology* 1985; 156:593-595.

Winzelberg GG, Froelich JW, McKusick KA, et al: Radionuclide localization of lower gastrointestinal hemorrhage. *Radiology* 1981; 139:465-469.

Winzelberg GG, McKusick KA, Strauss HW, et al: Evaluation of gastrointestinal bleeding by red blood cells labeled in vivo with technetium-99m. *J Nucl Med* 1979; 20:1080-1086.

Winzelberg GG, McKusick KA, Froelich JW, et al: Detection of gastrointestinal bleeding with ^{99m}Tc-labeled red blood cells. *Semin Nucl Med* 1982; 12:139-146.

6

Genitourinary System Imaging

RENAL SCANNING
Anatomy

I. Kidneys lie retroperitoneally between T-11 and L-3. The lower poles are approximately 2 to 3 cm above iliac crest.
II. Average length 12 cm. Left kidney slightly larger than right.
III. Left kidney lies slightly higher than right. Note that in women, right kidney often more mobile and ptotic.
IV. Kidneys divided into cortex and medulla.
V. Cortex contains:
   A. Glomeruli.
   B. Proximal and distal convoluted tubules.
VI. Medulla.
   A. Remaining tubular segments are in medulla.
   B. Portion of medulla that extends from just below outer cortex down toward renal pelvis—pyramids.
   C. Cortical projections between pyramids—columns of Bertin.

Physiology

I. Blood supply.
   A. Main renal artery, rarely duplicated. Branch into segmental arteries to arcuate to interlobar arteries and finally to glomeruli.
   B. Drugs may be excreted via:
      1. Glomerular filtration.
         a. Blood enters glomerulus through afferent arteriole. Filtration occurs. Filtrate moves into Bowman's capsule and into proximal convoluted tubule.
         b. Glomerular filtration rate (GFR) is number of milliliters of blood completely cleared of material in 1 minute.
         c. Normals—125 ml/minute.
      2. Proximal convoluted tubule function.
         a. Urine filtrate radically altered in proximal convoluted tubule (PCT). Most of H_2O reabsorbed plus Na^+, Cl^-, and HCO_3^-. In addition, glucose, amino acids, etc., all resorbed.

b. Note that materials have transport maximum.

c. In addition to resorption, many drugs, including hippuran, actively secreted here.

3. Loops of Henle.

a. Electrolytes resorbed, water not.

4. Distal convoluted tubule.

a. Resorption of sodium under hormonal control—antidiuretic hormone (ADH) or angiotensin system.

5. Collecting system—final part of system.

6. Arterial blood pressure affects tubular function. Results in prolonged intrarenal transit time of hippuran in renal artery stenosis.

Radiopharmaceuticals

I. Glomerular filtration rate agents.

A. To measure GFR accurately, radiopharmaceutical must:

1. Be completely filtered by glomerulus.

2. Not be protein bound (can't be filtered completely if it is).

3. Not be resorbed nor secreted by renal tubules.

4. Be excreted only by kidney (so that plasma sampling techniques, rather than urine sampling, can be used).

B. ^{99m}Tc diethylenetriamine pentaacetic acid (DTPA).

1. Soluble molecule, a chelate with a molecular weight of 500.

2. Meets requirement for measuring GFR *except* 3% to 5% protein bound. Percentage varies with different preparations. Protein binding causes false lowering of estimated GFR rates. Note that protein binding as low as 3% may cause significant error. More accurate estimates of GFR obtained when degree of protein binding in each specimen is measured and appropriate corrections made (or agent that does not bind plasma proteins is used).

3. After IV injection, rapidly penetrates capillary walls entering extracellular fluid by 3.8 minutes. DTPA does not enter cells because of lipid insolubility and negative charge.

4. Plasma disappearance—three components with half-times of 10, 90, 600 minutes, respectively, by 2 hours less than 10% injected dose in blood.

5. Normal renal filtration fraction (GFR divided by effective renin plasma flow) = 20%. Due to some protein binding, somewhat less than 20% of dose extracted.

6. Note that DTPA is completely eliminated by glomerular filtration; no tubular secretion occurs.

7. Originally, ferrous iron used to reduce pertechnetate for binding. Attempts to accelerate reduction by adding ascorbate

created complex that becomes cortically bound, not a GFR agent.

8. Quality control.
   a. ^{99m}Tc DTPA rapidly oxidized to pertechnetate by atmospheric oxygen. Problem with virtually all technetium pharmaceuticals.
   b. Insufficient tin may result in pertechnetate formation.
   c. Determination of quality via chromatographic techniques.
      (1) Hydrolyzed reduced Tc—immobility in aqueous or organic solvents.
      (2) Pertechnetate—mobile in organic solvents.

C. Chromium 51 EDTA.
1. Does not appear to have significant protein binding. Even so, gives GFR values slightly lower than inulin.

D. ^{125}I/^{131}I iothalamate.
1. Radiographic contrast agent.
2. Fifteen percent to 25% plasma protein bound.
3. Good correlation with inulin may come from cancellation of errors.

E. ^{131}I diatrizoate.
1. Radiographic contrast agent—Hypaque.

II. Tubular agents.

A. Ideal agent for measuring effective renal plasma flow (ERPF).
1. Totally removed from renal arterial blood during transit through kidney.
2. Volume of distribution should exceed plasma volume as little as possible, accelerating rate of excretion.
3. Protein binding not important if dissociation is rapid and does not affect extraction fraction. In fact, may be helpful by reducing volume of distribution.

B. ^{131}I orthoiodohippurate (OIH).
1. Chemically similar to paraaminohippuric acid (PAH). PAH is gold standard for measurement of renal plasma flow.
2. Prepared from conjugation of glycine with orthoiodobenzoic acid. Radiochemical contaminants are ^{131}I iodide and ^{131}I orthobenzoic acid. ^{131}I iodide can also be formed by autoradiolysis during storage. Both can lead to inaccurate ERPF, because both cleared more slowly than OIH. In fact, acid requires conjugation with glycine in liver to form OIH before excretion. Free iodide should be kept to less than 1.5% for accurate ERPF determination.
3. OIH extracted from blood by:
   a. Tubular secretion—80%.
   b. Glomerular filtration—20%.

4. Clearance of OIH dependent on:
    a. Renal blood flow.
    b. Renal extraction efficiency for OIH.
5. Ninety-six percent OIH extracted from renal arterial blood.
6. Sixty-six percent OIH bound to plasma proteins. Binding greater than for PAH. Remaining unbound fractions subject to glomerular filtration.
7. Red cells take up OIH; red cell concentration equals one-third total concentration of plasma. Rate of exchange between plasma and red cells is slow. Shifts are not enough to significantly affect measured plasma concentration significantly. Therefore, separation of plasma from red cells not required when measuring renal plasma flow.
8. Following IV injection, equilibrates with second space (extracellular space) over initial 4 to 5 minutes.
9. Intrarenal transit time—2.3 minutes.
10. Seventy percent injected dose excreted in urine—30 minutes.
11. Agent excreted without metabolic change.
12. Maximum concentration reached—2.5 to 3.4 minutes following injection.
13. Disappearance of agent from plasma is biexponential with fast and slow components. Fast component reflects intravascular renal clearance; slow component reflects clearance from interstitial space.

C. Technetium 99m mercaptoacetyltriglycine (MAG$_3$).
   1. Developed as a ^{99m}Tc replacement for ^{131}I OIH.
       a. Use of ^{99m}Tc.
           (1) 140 keV photon improves image quality compared to 364 keV photon of ^{131}I.
           (2) Lack of particulate emission (beta particle with ^{131}I) allows higher dose of MAG$_3$ to be used, further improving image quality and allowing flow study to be performed.
   2. Like OIH, MAG$_3$ excreted primarily by proximal convoluted tubules and not retained in kidney parenchyma.
   3. Differences from OIH.
       a. Glomerular filtration is 10%, compared to 20% for OIH.
       b. Plasma clearance is 70% of OIH, due to:
           (1) Higher protein binding (80% for MAG$_3$ vs 40% for OIH), which reduces amount of MAG$_3$ available for glomular filtration and tubular secretion.
           (2) Lower affinity for tubular transport mechanism than OIH.

(3) MAG$_3$ occasionally secreted through hepatobiliary system, leading to visualization of liver, bile ducts and gallbladder, and bowel. Seen most commonly in renal failure patients and may be due to impurities in preparation.

4. Even though plasma clearance is lower for MAG$_3$, it is proportional to OIH, which allows clearance of MAG$_3$ to be converted through regression formulas to ERPF calculated with OIH.

5. Renogram curves and rate at which two tracers appear in urine are essentially identical, even with difference in clearance.
   a. MAG$_3$, being more highly protein-bound, has a smaller volume of distribution than OIH, making it more available for secretion.
   b. Additionally, MAG$_3$ has less red cell uptake than OIH, also increasing amount of radiopharmaceutical available for excretion.

6. Preparation technique (US formulation).
   a. Sodium pertechnetate added to MAG$_3$ vial.
   b. 2 ml of filtered air added (air consumes any residual stannous ion, thereby increasing stability of preparation).
   c. Heated for 10 minutes in boiling water.
   d. Radiochemical purity 95% to 97%.
   e. Preparation stable for 6 hours after reconstitution.
   f. Note: European kit formulation is slightly different.
      (1) Radiochemical purity is lower (92% to 95%) with occasional yields as low as 80%.
      (2) Reconstituted kit has 1-hour expiration time limit.
      (3) Needs to be refrigerated after preparation.
      (4) Diluting individual doses three- or four-fold increases stability to 6 hours.

7. Dosimetry.
   a. ^{99m}Tc MAG$_3$ delivers a *lower* radiation dose per mCi than ^{131}I OIH, but it delivers a three to ten times *higher* absorbed radiation dose than ^{131}I OIH with clinical doses used, i.e., 10 mCi vs 300 µCi.
   b. In patients with renal failure or obstruction, however, ^{99m}Tc MAG$_3$ delivers significantly *lower* radiation dose than ^{131}I OIH.

8. Clinical comparisons with OIH and ^{99m}Tc DTPA.
   a. Quality of MAG$_3$ images superior to OIH in all patients.
   b. Quality of MAG$_3$ images especially superior to OIH and DTPA in renal failure patients.
   c. Findings on renal scan in various diseases usually identical between agents.

(1) MAG$_3$ and OIH have shown identical sensitivities and specificities in captopril renal imaging for renovascular hypertension.

(2) MAG$_3$ superior to OIH and DTPA in diuretic renography for obstruction due to superior image quality, especially in patients with diminished renal function.

III. Parenchymal agents.

A. Technetium 99m dimercaptosuccinic acid (DMSA).

1. Metal chelate used to treat heavy metal poisoning.

2. Following IV injection, 90% bound to plasma proteins—prevents significant glomerular filtration.

3. DMSA taken up into renal cortex (cortex/medullary ratio—22:1) in proximal convoluted tubule.

4. Renal extraction—4% to 5% per renal passage. 50% injected dose in kidneys within 1 hour. 50% still present in cortical tubules at 24 hours. 4% to 8% dose excreted in urine in 1 hour; 30% extracted by 14 hours. Note slow clearance related to degree of protein binding.

5. DMSA molecule splits upon reaching kidney. One moiety binds to renal tubules, other excreted.

6. In addition to renal uptake, hepatic uptake also seen. Varies with degree of renal function.

7. Gallbladder and gut may also be seen in renal failure.

8. Preparation unstable. Must be used within 30 minutes after preparation. Introduction of air increases instability; therefore, all doses should be drawn immediately from vial. Decreased renal uptake and increased liver uptake seen with breakdown of bond.

9. Note that acidification of the urine results in similar findings.

10. Urine excretion rate so low, collecting system not seen on images.

11. Usual dose—1 to 5 mCi.

12. Radiation—0.62 rad/mCi to kidney.

13. Note that dehydration produces decreased kidney-to-liver ratio. Important to maintain adequate hydration.

B. ^{99m}Tc glucoheptonate (glucose monocarboxylic acid).

1. Following IV injection, half plasma activity bound to protein. Excreted by:

a. Glomerular filtration.

b. Tubular extraction.

c. Ten percent remains bound to renal tubules at 1 to 2 hours.

d. Thus, does not reflect GFR or ERPF.

2. Approximately one half of dose excreted in urine in first 120

minutes (38% in urine within first hour). Thus, when imaged early can see collecting system; when imaged late, good cortical imaging.

3. As with agents secreted by tubules, some secretion into bile and gallbladder occasionally seen.
4. Most commonly used in pediatric patients.

C. Chlormerodrin Hg 191/203.

1. Mercurial diuretic. Radioactive mercury substituted for cold mercury.
2. Chlormerodrin Hg 203—beta emitter with 46.9-day half-life; chlormerodrin Hg 197—pure gamma emitter with 65-hour half-life.
3. 95% protein bound. Penetrates red cells reversibly.
4. Binds in proximal convoluted tubules. Plasma extraction slow, 10% to 20%.
5. Unlike other major renal radiopharmaceuticals—chlormerodrin is neutral.
6. Not currently used in clinical practice.

D. ^{99m}Tc penicillamine.

1. Behaves similarly to chlormerodrin and DMSA.
2. Because no advantages over DMSA, DMSA more commonly used.

Technique

I. Imaging.

A. Flow study.

1. Ten to 15 mCi of ^{99m}Tc DTPA or ^{99m}Tc GH, or 5 to 10 mCi of MAG$_3$, are injected in bolus.
2. Rapid sequential images are obtained every 2 seconds for 30 to 60 seconds.
3. Blood pool study may be obtained at this point.

B. Excretion studies.

1. The patient should be adequately hydrated unless examination is for hypertension, then some feel patient should be dehydrated. The patient should void before the study. A full bladder can simulate upper tract obstruction on the scan.
2. The patient is placed in a supine or prone position. Upright often causes the anterior displacement of superior pole of the kidney, foreshortening it. For hypertensive study, some position the patient in sitting position.
3. 150 to 300 µCi of ^{131}I OIH or 0.75 to 1 mCi of ^{123}I OIH is administered IV. For DTPA or other ^{99m}Tc agents, same dose used as for flow study.

4. Serial 3-minute images are obtained every 30 minutes.
5. All information is also stored on computer.
6. If drainage of material is delayed, the patient is asked to re-void and walk around. A second set of images is then obtained. This will help distinguish obstruction from dilatation or slow-flow situations.

C. Static imaging.
1. Glucoheptonate.
   a. Early imaging such as with DTPA reveals the collecting system.
   b. Delayed imaging—2 to 3 hours for cortex.
2. DMSA.
   a. Two- to 3-hour delay.
   b. May delay imaging up to 24 hours if patient in severe renal failure.
   c. This allows slow extraction to occur, decreasing background.

D. Determination of GFR.
1. Clearance is:
   a. $C = UV/P$ where C = clearance in ml/minute; U = concentration of indicator per milliliter; V = ml of urine excreted/minute; and P = plasma concentration per milliliter.
   b. In other words, if substance has plasma concentration of 1 mg/ml, urine excretion of 100 mg/min, then 100 ml of plasma cleared per minute = GFR.
   c. By continuous IV infusion, adjusted so that plasma level remains constant over period of study.
   d. Urine collections at 20 minutes each, three times, can be performed.
   e. This classical technique has been used with inulin, a fructose polymer from plant sources for measuring GFR. It may also be used with radioactive materials.
2. Sapirstein technique.
   a. Use concept of compartmental analysis (see below).

$$
\begin{array}{l}
\text{Injection} \\
V_1 \rightarrow v_2 \\
\downarrow \\
V_3
\end{array}
$$

V_1 = theoretical volume including plasma volume; V_2 = closed system in which material equilibrates; identity is not clear but represents essentially extravascular space; V_3 = kidney-urine.

    b. Multiple plasma samples are obtained and counts are plotted vs. time on semilog paper.

    c. A biexponential curve is found with a fast and slow component. The fast component represents intravascular renal clearance; slow component reflects clearance from interstitial space. The slow component (λa) is subtracted from the curve deriving the fast component (λb), and the intercepts of A and B along the Y axis (counts per minute) are determined. GFR then equals

$$\frac{I \times a\lambda \; b\lambda}{(A \times \lambda b) \; 1 \; (B \times \lambda a)}$$

where I = total radioactivity injected

$$\text{Using half-times GFR} = \frac{I \times 0.693}{(A \times t^{1/2}a) \; 1 \; (B \times t^{1/2}b)}$$

3. Single sample.

    a. Plasma disappearance rate is generally proportional to blood flow to kidney.

    b. While early portion of plasma disappearance curve reflects intercompartmental shifts, terminal segment of curve is assumed to bear closer relation to GFR.

    c. Points on the curve were examined to find if one might correlate sufficiently well with GFR to be used to measure GFR.

    d. Optimum sampling time depends on GFR.

       (1) 100 ml/minute or greater—120 minutes.

       (2) 60 to 100 ml/minute—150 minutes.

       (3) <60 ml/minute—220 minutes.

4. Two-sample protein-free plasma clearance method.

    a. Correlates extremely well with gold standard of ^{125}I iothalamate.

    b. Technique.

       (1) Prepare two equal aliquots 3 mCi of ^{99m}Tc DTPA.

       (2) Inject one dose; use other as standard.

       (3) Draw blood into EDTA anticoagulated tubes at 60 and 180 minutes in opposite arm to the one injected with original dose.

       (4) Centrifuge at 2000 rpm for 10 minutes and remove plasma.

       (5) Centrifuge plasma in Centrifree micropartition tubes at 2000 rpm for 15 minutes to obtain plasma-free fluid.

       (6) Count duplicate aliquots of samples and equal volume of standard dilution in gamma well counter.

(7) Calculate GFR.

(8) $GFR = [(D \; Ln(P_1/P_2)/(T_1 - T_2)) \times e^{((T_1 LnP_2 - T_2 LnP_1)/(T_2 - T_1))}]^{0.979}$

where:

D = Dose activity, counts/minute.

T_1 = Time of collection of first blood sample in minutes (60).

T_2 = Time of collection of second blood sample (180).

P_1 = Ultrafiltrate activity (in cpm/ml) at $T_1 \times 0.94$.

P_2 = Ultrafiltrate activity (in cpm/ml) at $T_2 \times 0.94$.

5. Imaging computer technique.
    a. Gates adapted Schlegel technique for ERPF (see below).
    b. Corrected uptake of ^{99m}Tc DTPA during 2 to 3 minutes after injection used via regression equation determined from studies comparing corrected renal uptakes in DTPA with creatinine clearance GFR.
    c. Note that relative GFR can be determined by percentage counts in region of interest of left kidney (after background subtraction) divided by left plus right kidney.
    d. Normal GFR = 125 ml/minute.
E. Determination of effective renal plasma flow (ERPF).
    1. ERPF.
        a. "Effective" indicates that flow to capsule-interstitial tissues is excluded.
        b. "Plasma" indicates only plasma activity is assayed with technique.
    2. Techniques based on same theoretical considerations as GFR in previous section.
        a. Clearance technique.
        b. Multiple sample—Sapirstein's technique.
        c. Single sample.
            (1) Close correlations between concentration reciprocal (injected dose counts divided by plasma counts) instead of usual plasma counts divided by dose counts, when plasma samples were obtained 44.5 minutes after injection. Error of ERPF with single plasma sample is ±30 ml/min.
        d. Imaging-computer technique.
            (1) Schlegel technique.
            (2) Renal uptake based on premise that renal uptake of ^{131}I OIH in first 1 to 2 minutes following injection reflects total ERPF to each kidney.
            (3) Renal radioactivity is corrected for:

(a) Dose injected.
(b) Attenuation—distance of kidneys from camera.
(c) Background.

(4) Corrected renal uptake is

$$\frac{(1\text{- to 2-min kidney counts} - \text{background counts} \times Y^2) \times 100}{1\text{-min counts injected}}$$

where Y = kidney depth in centimeters as determined by ratio of weight to height.

(5) Percentage return.
  (a) Percentage of injected dose of OIH recovered in urine in 30 minutes after correction for residual bladder activity.
  (b) Fractional excretion of 68% or greater is considered normal.
  (c) Schlegel has related this number to ERPF via regression equation.

(6) Normal ERPF = 500 to 600 ml/minute.
(7) ERPF is *not* affected by hydration state of patient.
(8) Contamination with 3% to 5% free ^{131}I produces errors of up to 25% on ERPF.
(9) OIH calculated ERPF usually 10% below PAH levels. Differences may result from:
  (a) Inhibition by PAH in macrochemical concentrations when both were performed simultaneously.
  (b) Presence of unrecognized contaminates (i.e., ^{131}I).
  (c) Localized protein or cellular binding.
  (d) Differences in handling of two agents by kidney.

F. Filtration fraction (FF) = GFR divided by ERPF. Normal is 0.2. When FF is abnormal, it is usually high and indicates tubular function more seriously disrupted than glomerular function. In fact, in most disease states, ERPF is more sensitive than GFR in detecting abnormalities. FF increases with decreased plasma protein or congestive heart failure. FF decreases because of decline in GFR in glomerulonephritis, for example.

G. Intrarenal transit time.
  1. Using deconvolution (a mathematical process), the continuous input of hippuran can be seen as a single bolus injection into the renal artery. Curve obtained by deconvolution is called impulse retention function.
  2. Excretion index (EI) may also be calculated in a more simple manner. This reflects transit time.
  3. EI equals percent dose voided plus percent dose residual (bladder) divided by percent dose expected in patient.

a. Note that by use of mathematical equations, possibility exists to predict percentage injected dose that should be in excretory tract. This reflects transit time as well as tubular function and filtration fraction.

Normal Scan

I. Renal flow study.
   A. Both kidneys visualize symmetrically and with similar intensities. The intensity of a kidney of normal size should equal or exceed the early activity in spleen.
   B. Slope of curve of activity entering each kidney should parallel aortic flow curves. Peak should occur no more than 3 seconds later than aortic peak.
   C. Splenic and liver activity may simulate kidney activity.
   D. Bowel "blush" in nephrectomy site may simulate renal perfusion.
II. Excretory phase.
   A. Prompt uptake of material with peak at approximately 3 to 5 minutes and then declining activity.
   B. Renal pelvis/bladder activity usually seen in 3 to 6 minutes.
   C. Upstrokes of two kidneys are parallel—heights vary by kidney size. Downslope may vary depending on variations in collecting systems. Dilated or slower draining, but not obstructed, collecting systems will show slower transit. Imaging after voiding in upright position should help differentiate from obstruction. Late images also useful.
   D. Increased spleen and especially liver activity may be seen in face of renal failure.
   E. When renal function is poor, vicarious excretion may occur via GI tract. Gallbladder or colon may be seen.
   F. With dehydration, a curve may resemble obstruction.
   G. Normal:
      1. GFR—125 ml/minute.
      2. ERPF—500 to 600 ml/minute.
      3. Filtration fraction—0.2.
      4. Excretory index—1.
III. Static images.
   A. Smooth renal contour.
   B. Note: Normally, defects are seen due to collecting system and irregularities at corticomedullary junction.

Abnormal Scan

I. Vascular disease.
   A. Renovascular hypertension
      1. Background.

a. Hypertension affects 60 million Americans.
b. Hypertensive cardiovascular disease is a leading cause of death in the U.S.
c. Renovascular hypertension is major potentially curable form of hypertension.
d. Advances in noninvasive testing have been stimulated by advances in PTCA and surgical techniques to correct renovascular hypertension.
e. Prevalence of renovascular hypertension is approximately 0.5%—considerably lower than earlier estimates of 5%.
   (1) Low prevalence makes it important to perform renal scans on patients who are moderate- or high-risk, based on clinical criteria, to maintain adequate specificity.
      (a) If screening were performed on all hypertensive patients, only 1 of 200 would actually have renovascular hypertension; thus, even using a noninvasive screening test that has a sensitivity and specificity of 90%, almost all positive cases would be false-positives.
   (2) Groups have recommended testing patients with 5% to 15% to 50% probabilities of renovascular hypertension. Some hypertensive experts believe patients with a high likelihood of renovascular hypertension should proceed directly to angiography, without noninvasive tests.
f. Clinical criteria for selecting patients to be tested recommended by the Working Group for Patient Selection and Preparation—Captopril Renogram Consensus Conference include (but are not necessarily limited to) patients with:
   (1) Onset of hypertension (diastolic blood pressure ≥105 mm Hg) in individuals ≤25 years of age.
   (2) Recent onset of hypertension, especially if diastolic blood pressure ≥105 mm Hg.
   (3) Hypertension that cannot be brought under control with adequate antihypertensive drug regimen.
   (4) Longstanding, well-controlled hypertension who become refractory to their existing medications.
   (5) Hypertension and abdominal bruits, especially if long and in the region of the renal artery.
   (6) Hypertension and generalized vascular occlusive disease (peripheral vascular, coronary, cerebrovascular).
   (7) Hypertension and elevated creatinine in which no

other etiology for renal failure is present.

    (8) New or more severe renal failure when treated with angiotensin-converting enzyme (ACE) inhibitors.

  g. Note: Criteria above are regardless of race; however, hypertension has much higher prevalence in blacks compared to whites (18.5% vs 6.7%). In addition, the incidence of severe hypertension (diastolic of 115 mm Hg or greater) is eight times higher in blacks; however, the incidence of renovascular hypertension, even in patients with suggestive clinical clues, is two to three times lower than in whites.

  h. Note: In addition to using above criteria, clinical judgment is also used to select who is tested. Recent onset of hypertension of 150/100 mm Hg might provoke noninvasive testing if patient had previously been consistently running BPs of 100/70 mm Hg.

2. Causes.

  a. Fibromuscular dysplasia often associated with primary ptosis of right kidney further compromising lumen of affected kidney when patient upright.

    (1) 80% in women.

    (2) Average age, 30 to 40 years.

    (3) Usually a right-sided lesion.

    (4) Lesions consist of one or more fibrous or fibromuscular cusps with poststenotic dilatation. These areas are prone to dissection.

  b. Atherosclerotic disease.

    (1) Occurs primarily in males 60 years or older.

    (2) Usually bilateral. Caused by plaques at origin or in course of renal arteries.

  c. Both types may result in arterial hypertension caused by release of renin from juxtaglomular apparatus as result of anoxia, pressure changes, or lower sodium in distal tubules. Renin cleaves angiotensinogen produced in liver to angiotensin I. This further cleaved in lung to angiotensin II, the most potent vasoconstrictor known.

  d. Stenotic lesion may result in diminished pressure at glomerulus, resulting in dampening of normal renal artery pulsations and reduced glomerular filtration. This results in increased water and sodium resorption, diminished urine volume, and increased osmolality.

3. Physiology.

  a. Constriction of a main renal artery leads to cascade of

events involving renin-angiotensin-aldosterone system (RAAS).

b. Initial vasodilatation of main renal artery distal to stenosis occurs in attempt to maintain renal blood flow.

c. This causes decreased renal perfusion pressure resulting in decreased glomerular filtration rate (GFR).

d. Decreased perfusion pressure stimulates renin release from juxtaglomerular apparatus of affected kidney.

e. Renin stimulates conversion of angiotensinogen > angiotensin I.

f. Angiotensin-converting enzyme (ACE) converts decapeptide angiotensin I > octopeptide angiotensin II.

g. Angiotensin II has two primary effects:
   (1) Causes renal vasoconstriction with preferential glomerular efferent arteriolar constriction, maintaining glomerular filtration rate.
   (2) Stimulates release of aldosterone with sodium retention.

h. Captopril is an ACE inhibitor; it:
   (1) Eliminates angiotensin II-induced glomerular arteriolar vasoconstriction.
   (2) Causes decreased GFR, urine flow, and salt retention in affected kidney.
   (3) This is basis of captopril renal scan. In the kidney with renal artery stenosis, a decrease in renal function is seen after captopril administration.

4. Technique.
   a. Study usually performed in two parts:
      (1) First, a routine (pre-captopril) renal scan is performed.
      (2) Second, 4 to 48 hours later, a second scan is performed after administration of captopril (post-captopril study). Changes in function between pre-captopril and post-captopril scan are used for diagnosis of renovascular hypertension.
   b. Patient preparation.
      (1) Captopril is discontinued for 2 days. Longer-acting agents such as lisinopril and enalopril are discontinued for 7 days.
      (2) Some groups discontinue diuretics for 1 to 3 days to reduce risk of severe blood pressure falls with ACE-inhibition. Others leave patients on diuretics.
      (3) Oral hydration is encouraged before study.

c. Choice of radiopharmaceutical.
  (1) ^{99m}Tc DTPA—10 to 20 mCi.
    (a) Advantages.
      (i) A glomerular agent; good photon flux yields high-quality images.
      (ii) Allows quantification of GFR.
  (2) I-131 hippuran—300 μCi.
    (a) Advantages.
      (i) Excreted by both glomerular filtration and tubular secretion.
      (ii) Very high extraction ratio and excretion, making it superior to DTPA in patients with poor baseline renal function.
      (iii) Allows quantification of ERPF.
    (b) Disadvantage.
      (i) Poor photon flux with ^{131}I yields poor-quality images.
  (3) Combined DTPA and hippuran.
    (a) Perform 10 mCi ^{99m}Tc DTPA renal scan followed immediately by 300 μCi ^{131}I hippuran scan.
    (b) Advantage.
      (i) Combines best of both radiopharmaceuticals.
    (c) Disadvantages.
      (i) More expensive and time-consuming.
  (4) ^{99m}Tc MAG$_3$—3 to 10 mCi.
    (a) Advantages.
      (i) Combines ^{99m}Tc labeling and physiologic handling similar to hippuran.
      (ii) Works well in patients with diminished renal function.
    (b) Disadvantage.
      (i) Does not allow direct GFR or ERPF measurement; however, can use regression analysis formula to yield hippuran-equivalent ERPF.
d. Pre-captopril renal scan.
  (1) Perform flow and function studies.
  (2) ^{99m}Tc DTPA technique (include GFR measurement).
  (3) ^{131}I hippuran technique (include ERPF measurement).
    (a) Note: Some investigators give 20 mg lasix at 3 minutes during hippuran phase to reduce collecting system activity, which might be misinterpreted as cortical retention.
  (4) Combined DTPA and hippuran technique (include ERPF measurement).

        (a) Note: Some investigators give 20 mg lasix at 3 minutes during hippuran phase to reduce collecting system activity, which might be misinterpreted as cortical retention.

     (5) ^{99m}Tc MAG$_3$ technique. (Include numeric function measurement.)

  e. Post-captopril study.

     (1) Blood pressure measured at baseline and every 10 to 15 minutes thereafter.

     (2) Patient is given 25 to 50 mg captopril orally.

     (3) One hour later, renal scan is performed using same protocol and radiopharmaceutical as for pre-captopril study.

     (4) Some institutions perform post-captopril scan first; if it is normal, study is stopped.

5. Interpretation.

  a. Working Party on Diagnostic Criteria of Renovascular Hypertension with Captopril Renography recommends semi-quantitative approach. Each kidney is graded on scan as follows:

     (1) Grade 0—normal.

     (2) Grade 1—any one of the following:

        (a) Mild delay in upslope.

        (b) Decreased maximal activity.

        (c) Abnormal T_{max} (time to maximal activity), $6 \le T_{max} \le 11$ minutes.

        (d) Delayed excretory phase, but downsloping.

     (3) Grade 2A.

        (a) Delay in upstroke and T_{max} *with* an excretory phase.

     (4) Grade 2B.

        (a) Delay in upslope and T_{max} *without* an excretory phase.

     (5) Grade 3.

        (a) Marked reduction or absence of uptake.

     (6) Scans are interpreted as:

        (a) High-probability for renovascular hypertension—a change of one grade or more (including 2A > 2B) between pre- and post-captopril.

        (b) Low-probability—Grade 0 post-captopril.

        (c) Indeterminate—abnormal baseline scan, which does not change between the pre- and post-captopril scans. Note: Grade 2B or 3 scans that do not change are especially worrisome; Grade 1s are less so. However, nonrenovascular intrinsic renal disease *cannot* be differentiated from renovascular hypertension with this pattern.

  (d) Additional, more quantitative, criteria for interpretation are sometimes used. These include:
   (i) Change in split function (60/40% or greater ratio).
   (ii) Parenchymal transit time.
   (iii) Residual cortical activity (counts at 20 to 30 minutes vs peak counts).
   (iv) Change in measured total GFR (15% fall or greater).
      a Especially useful for detecting bilateral renal artery stenosis and in patients with only one kidney.

6. Accuracy.
  a. Sensitivity and specificity depend on patient population studied and specific criteria used to interpret scans.
   (1) Averge sensitivity and specificity of test in three recent studies (205 patients with 46% prevalence of renovascular hypertension): sensitivity 93%, specificity 95%.
   (2) European Captopril Radionuclide Test Multicenter Study Group (424 patients with 54% prevalence of renovascular hypertension):
    (a) Sensitivity.
     (i) Unilateral renal artery stenosis—73%.
     (ii) Bilateral renal artery stenosis—91%.
    (b) Specificity.
     (i) Overall—84%.
     (ii) Patients without renal insufficiency—92%.

7. Special considerations.
  a. Bilateral renal artery stenosis.
   (1) Twenty-nine percent of patients with renovascular hypertension have bilateral stenoses.
   (2) Asymmetric involvement usually exists so that captopril study shows asymmetric changes in function between pre- and post-captopril renal scans.
   (3) It can be difficult to appreciate whether the more functional kidney is also involved.
  b. Branch stenosis.
   (1) Can be missed with captopril renal scan study.
  c. Transplant renal artery stenosis.

        (1) Transplant renal artery stenosis causes 5% of post-transplant hypertension.

        (2) Captopril useful though not as reliable in single-kidney model.

B. Renal artery embolism.

  1. Background.

    a. Embolism most common cause of major renal vascular occlusion; in situ thrombosis accounts for only 4% of renal infarction.

    b. Cardiac lesions constitute primary site of embolization. Subacute bacterial endocarditis (SBE) and rheumatic heart disease with fibrillating atria most common cardiac lesions.

    c. Bilateral involvement in 50% of cases.

    d. Clinical picture consists of sudden onset of flank pain with asociated hematuria and anuria.

  2. Findings.

    a. Absent flow.

    b. Absent function.

C. Renal vein thrombosis.

  1. Background.

    a. Most frequently occurs in infants because of dehydration.

    b. May occur in adults because of hypercoagulability, post-surgery, or obstruction of renal blood flow due to tumor, lymphadenopathy, etc.

  2. Findings.

    a. Decreased flow.

    b. Enlarged kidney. May be normal size if thrombosis incomplete or slowly developing or long-standing.

    c. Prolonged parenchymal transit time.

II. Renal trauma.

A. Findings.

  1. Renal artery injury/occlusion.

    a. No evidence of flow.

    b. No evidence of function.

  2. Segmental renal infarction.

    a. Decreased function in region of kidney that will not improve over a period of weeks.

  3. Renal contusion.

    a. Decreased function in a portion of kidney. Function will return over a matter of weeks.

  4. Renal rupture/fracture.

    a. Disruption of normal renal outline on delayed imaging.

      5. Urinary extravasation.
        a. Activity outside normal confines of ureter/bladder.
      6. Arteriovenous fistula.
        a. Complication of renal biopsy or penetrating trauma.
        b. Flow study reveals more rapid filling of abnormal vascular channel than remainder of kidney. Rapid visualization of venous system.
      7. Perirenal hematoma.
        a. Unilateral decreased perfusion.

III. Renal inflammation/infection.
   A. Acute pyelonephritis.
      1. Clinical findings.
        a. Pyuria.
        b. Costovertebral pain and tenderness.
        c. Intravenous pyelogram (IVP) positive in only 25%.
        d. Studies with radionuclides almost always abnormal.
      2. Scan findings.
        a. Multiple, frequently bilateral, photopenic defects. These have indistinct margins that appear to flare from pelvocalyceal structures to renal periphery.
        b. Note that flow study may show diminished perfusion in same regions. If infection spreads into perirenal space, there may be decreased perfusion of entire kidney due to tamponade.
   B. Chronic pyelonephritis.
      1. Findings.
        a. Similar to acute pyelonephritis. In addition, evidence of decreased size and scarring may be seen.
        b. Function may appear decreased. Note that chronic pyelonephritis is most common cause of unilateral renal atrophy. Other conditions that must be considered in unilateral atrophy include:
          (1) Postobstructive atrophy.
          (2) Renal artery stenosis.
          (3) Congenital hypoplasia.
          (4) Renal infarction.
          (5) Radiation atrophy.
          (6) Tuberculosis.
   C. Renal abscess/carbuncle.
      1. Findings.
        a. Similar to focal pyelonephritis except that blood flow images may demonstrate increased activity in some cases.
   D. Radiation nephritis.

1. Can occur with as little as 1,500 rad over 2½ weeks.
2. Generalized or focally decreased activity depending on how much of kidney was included in radiation portal. Sharp straight borders of involved area may be seen at edge of treatment field—helps make diagnosis.
3. Increased uptake of bone agents has been described in acute phase.
E. Acute interstitial nephritis.
1. Patients may show increased gallium uptake. Note that ATN has occasionally been associated with uptake as well.
IV. Obstructive uropathy.
A. Urinary calculi are most common cause of obstruction. Majority pass spontaneously. Other causes of postrenal obstruction include:
1. Inflammation.
2. Neurogenic effects.
3. Neoplasm.
4. Thrombi.
5. Congenital disorders.
B. Bilateral obstruction usually caused by lower tract obstruction.
C. High-grade obstruction of only 1 week's duration can produce permanent decrease in renal function.
D. Glomerular function is compromised by obstruction earlier than tubular function. In fact, when obstruction is partial, the renal parenchyma is well preserved and ERPF is normal or paradoxically increased. For these reasons, tubular agents are often recommended over GFR agents in obstruction.
E. Findings.
1. Delayed and diminished blood flow to involved side (acute obstruction).
2. Delayed cortical visualization.
3. Prolonged transit time.
4. Hang-up and dilatation of collecting system.
5. Nonvisualization of bladder in cases of bilateral complete obstruction.
6. With long-standing or complete obstruction, nonvisualization of kidney may occur. Note that even in kidneys with nonvisualization, recovery may occur.
7. Note that blood flow may be diminished in nonobstructed dilatation in proportion to parenchymal damage that may have occurred from previous obstruction. However, delay does not occur.
8. With cortical areas of interest excluding collecting system, normal cortical curves may be obtained. This indicates func-

tion of kidney well preserved. In cases in which it is unclear whether patient is obstructed or has dilated or atonic collecting system, delayed views are helpful. Obstruction will not drain, whereas dilated nonobstructed collecting systems will.

9. Static imaging agents such as DMSA appear to overestimate degree of function in an acute obstruction.

F. Diuretic renogram.
  1. Background.
    a. Whitaker test—gold standard for diagnosing obstruction.
      (1) Percutaneous puncture of collecting system performed.
      (2) Fluid infused at known rate and pressure in system is measured; resistance can then be calculated.
      (3) Disadvantages.
        (a) Invasive.
        (b) Unreliable in large-volume hydroureteronephrosis.
    b. Diuretic renogram.
      (1) Physiologic bolus of urine generated by administration of diuretic; clearance of radiopharmaceutical is then monitored.
        (a) Advantages.
          (i) Noninvasive.
          (ii) Quantitative.
          (iii) Measures renal function.
      (2) Technique—developed by Consortium of Pediatric Nuclear Medicine Club (Society of Nuclear Medicine) and Society of Fetal Urology.
        (a) Patient preparation.
          (i) Delay study if possible until 1 month of age (later in a premature infant) to reduce likelihood of immature renal function from affecting results.
        (b) Hydration.
          (i) Oral hydration ad libitum 2 hours before study.
          (ii) Normal saline solution (D5.3 NS or D5.25 NS) at a rate to deliver 15 ml/kg over 30 minutes beginning at least 15 minutes before injection of radiopharmaceutical.
          (iii) Continue infusion during study at maintenance—200 ml/kg/24 hours.
        (c) If patient unable to void on command, if bladder

noncompliant, or if reflux is present, catheter should be placed in bladder.

2. Radiopharmaceutical.
   a. ^{99m}Tc MAG$_3$—50 mCi/kg (minimum 1 mCi).
3. Imaging procedure.
   a. Patient should be in prone position.
   b. Camera should be placed posteriorly.
   c. Use SFOV or LFOV camera—magnification might be necessary.
   d. Digital acquisition—20 seconds per frame (128 × 128 matrix).
   e. Analog acquisition—1 to 2 minutes/image for 50 minutes.
   f. Furosemide, 1 mg/kg in children, is given at 20 to 30 minutes or when entire collecting system is full. Increased time before injection is necessary if decreased renal function present, to allow collecting system to fill.
   g. In adults, 20 to 80 mg plus of furosemide is given, depending on renal function.
4. Data analysis.
   a. Renogram phase—ROI encompasses entire kidney, including renal pelvis. Background ROI—two pixels wide and circles kidney ROI.
   b. Diuretic phase—ROI encompasses renal pelvis only. Background ROI inferior and lateral to lower pole of kidney. Separate ureteral ROI is also done.
5. Interpretation.
   a. Many clinicians measure $T_{1/2}$ from the time furosemide is given:
      (1) 10 minutes—no obstruction.
      (2) 10 to 20 minutes—equivocal.
      (3) Greater than 20 minutes—obstruction.
   b. Others recommend using renogram and diuretic response patterns:
      (1) Normal—no obstruction.
      (2) Flat, or best if upsloping curve—obstruction.
      (3) Slow washout—indeterminate.
   c. Note: Split function is not useful; for unknown reasons, early after obstruction affected kidney usually has normal or increased measured split function.
   d. Problems:
      (1) Type of technique used is critical (hydration, data analysis, etc). Any variation of technique can lead to spurious findings.

(2) With decreased renal function, increased $T_{1/2}$ and poor or little washout is not uncommon; must be careful not to diagnose obstruction—these studies are indeterminate.

(3) With large-volume hydroureteronephrosis, there is a prolonged $T_{1/2}$ even without obstruction, due to a mixing chamber effect of the radiopharmaceutical in large static volume of nonradioactive urine.

(4) Compliance of collecting system and bladder are important.

    (a) Noncompliance of pelvis might result in "normal $T_{1/2}$."

    (b) Compliant collecting system might give decreased washout even without obstruction.

    (c) Noncompliant bladder or reflux can cause increased back pressure resulting in false-positive study.

V. Mass lesions.

  A. Tumor.

    1. Hypernephroma.

      a. Most common renal neoplasm in adults.

      b. Constitutes 85% of renal cancers.

      c. Maximum incidence sixth decade.

      d. May present as painless hematuria or symptoms related to metastatic foci in lungs, bone, and liver.

      e. Findings.

        (1) Increased flow.

        (2) Area of decreased activity on delayed imaging.

    2. Renal angiomyolipoma.

      a. Fifty percent to 80% of patients with tuberous sclerosis will have renal angiomyolipomas.

      b. Findings.

        (1) Due to rich vascularity, lesion seen on flow study.

        (2) Cold area on delayed imaging.

    3. Wilms' tumor.

      a. Constitutes 20% of childhood malignancies.

      b. Metastasizes to regional nodes, lung, brain, and liver.

    4. Pseudomasses on urogram.

      a. Hypertrophied Bertin's columns.

      b. Dromedary humps.

      c. Fetal lobulations.

      d. Splenic impressions.

      e. Findings.

(1) All are functional tissue. They show more intense uptake of renal agents than remainder of kidney because of greater thickness of parenchyma in these regions.

B. Cysts.
 1. Simple cysts.
    a. Common—asymptomatic. Usually small (<2.5 cm) situated in renal cortex.
    b. Lesions as small as 1 cm can be identified if peripheral. More central location requires larger size to be seen.
    c. Findings.
       (1) No evidence of increased flow; in fact, a photopenic area.
       (2) Cold area on delayed imaging.
 2. Polycystic disease.
    a. Infantile form—usually evident at, or shortly after, birth—leads to early death.
       (1) Rare—inherited as autosomal-recessive.
       (2) Associated with hepatic fibrosis and cysts of bile duct origin.
       (3) Hepatic dysfunction common.
    b. Adult form.
       (1) Familial—inherited as autosomal-dominant.
       (2) May be manifest in infancy—most commonly, however, develops in adulthood.
       (3) Approximately one third of patients will have associated polycystic disease of liver. No apparent impairment of liver function in most cases. Note approximately 50% of patients with polycystic disease of liver have associated polycystic disease of kidneys. Cysts may also be found in thyroid, pancreas, and other organs.
    c. Findings.
       (1) Multiple cold defects on scintigraphy.
 3. Medullary sponge kidney.
    a. Affects males twice as often as females.
    b. Appears in adults—usually does not affect life span.
    c. Seventy-five percent are bilateral.
    d. Cysts are small and tend to occur at tips of papillae. Unilateral cysts may be confined to single lobe.
    e. Clinically, patients complain of flank pain and "sandy" urine. May have recurrent infections.
    f. Findings.

           (1) ERPF mildly/severely depressed.

           (2) Transit time prolonged.

           (3) Function may be asymmetrical.

    4. Medullary cystic disease.

      a. Occurs in young adults.

      b. Cysts of 1 cm or less form in medulla of kidney—kidneys appear small and quite fibrotic. Eye diseases may occur in association with this disease.

      c. Findings.

           (1) Evidence of multiple cysts.

           (2) Decreased renal size.

VI. Anomalies of position and number.

  A. Renal ectopia.

    1. Occurs in men, usually involving left kidney. In migration, kidney loses reniform shape, becomes discoid or spherical.

    2. Crossed ectopia—one kidney crosses opposite side, caudal to normal kidney—85% of time migrating kidney fused to lower pole.

  B. Horseshoe kidney.

    1. Fusion occurs as a single band inferiorly, which may or may not contain functioning elements. The pelves are separate and rotated anteriorly. Ureters pass anteriorly across lower pole of kidneys.

    2. May be difficult to appreciate band of tissue because of non-function or spinal column attenuation. Anterior images may be useful.

  C. Unilateral agenesis.

    1. Usually involves left kidney.

  D. Supernumery kidneys.

    1. Rare.

    2. Small—lie caudal to normal kidney and drain independently into ipsilateral ureter or bladder.

    3. Increased risk of infection.

VII. Evaluation in acute and chronic renal failure.

  A. OIH—uptake sufficient for visualization with as little as 3% of normal function; 18 of 19 patients with blood urea nitrogen (BUN) levels ranging from 62 to 146 mg/dl and creatinine levels of 3.5 to 17.2 successfully imaged with hippuran.

  B. Technetium DTPA visualization can occur in patients with BUN levels over 65 mg/dl.

  C. Tubular agents superior to DTPA in uremia. DMSA probably best. Delayed imaging as long as 24 hours after injection is sometimes necessary for background to clear.

D. Note that increasing amount of liver activity seen with progressive renal failure. Especially seen with tubular agents and technetium cortical agents. Somewhat less prominent with glucoheptonate than DMSA. Hardly ever seen with DTPA.

E. Renal imaging in uremic patients more likely successful following hemodialysis when noncortical agents are used. This probably due to removal of competing organic anions in dialysis.

F. Renal imaging also better shortly after acute reduction of renal function than later after uremic solutes have accumulated.

G. Patients with chronic renal failure and lack of OIH uptake have poor prognosis.

H. Filtration fraction may be helpful.
   a. Increased in ATN.
   b. Decreased in prerenal states.
   c. Normal in postrenal obstruction.

TRANSPLANT EVALUATION

I. Background.
   A. Living related donor—90% chance of surviving 10 years. ATN almost never occurs.
   B. Cadaveric graft—ATN common postoperatively, may be related to warm ischemia time or changes in oxygenation or perfusion that occurred before donor's death.

II. Rejection.
   A. Hyperacute rejection.
      1. Due to presence of preformed antibodies in recipient's circulation because of loss of previous graft, multiple transfusions, or multiple pregnancies.
      2. Leads to rapid thrombosis of vascular bed and functional destruction within minutes to hours. Occurs within first 1 to 12 hours following rejection.
   B. Accelerated rejection.
      1. Predominantly cell-mediated—occurs earlier than acute rejection. Occurs 1 to 5 days after transplantation.
      2. Results from sensitization of recipient population.
   C. Acute rejection.
      1. Cell-mediated process. Sensitized lymphocytes migrate into graft and destroy cells *without* participation of humoral antibodies.
      2. Clinical signs.
         a. Fever.
         b. Renal enlargement.
         c. Tenderness of graft.

      d. Decreased urine output.

      e. Increased serum creatinine.

  D. Chronic rejection.

    1. Humoral antibody-induced injury to endothelial and interstitial cells. Causes narrowing of vascular bed, decreased renal size, hypertension, and ultimately renal failure.

    2. Irreversible.

Normal Scan

  I. Flow.

    A. Peak renal activity within 4 to 6 seconds of peak aortic activity. About equal to iliac activity.

    B. Maximal intensity of renal activity will equal or exceed aortic/iliac activity.

    C. Activity within kidney rapidly increases to clearly define maximum, then falls to lower levels.

    D. Various computer indices can also be used, including:

      1. Time to reach peak activity.

      2. Time to reach peak activity, then fall to one-half peak.

      3. Mean slope of upstroke of time-activity curve.

      4. Maximum slope of upstroke.

      5. Time interval of upstroke (area under the curve) of time-activity curve.

      6. In each instance, quantitative index of renal curve compared with same curve for aortic or iliac curve.

  II. Parenchymal imaging.

    A. Normal findings similar to those of native kidneys.

 III. Dehydration does not influence ERPF value. Average normal ERPF in transplanted kidney 350 ml/minute; range, 250 to 500 ml/minute.

Abnormal Scan

  I. Absence of flow and function—early.

    A. Causes.

      1. Renal artery occlusion.

      2. Renal vein thrombosis.

      3. Renal cortical necrosis.

  II. Acute tubular necrosis (ATN).

    A. Usually occurs within first 24 hours. Usually reaches maximum at 48 hours and then shows improvement. This is in distinction to rejection, which shows progressively worsening function without treatment.

    B. Flow.

      1. Much better preserved than one might suppose from diminished function.

C. Frequently no excretion from kidney is seen.
III. Acute rejection.
    A. Usually occurs after 5 days postoperatively; often occurs within first 3 months; can occur even later.
    B. Flow usually more affected than in ATN. Flow more closely follows decreased function.
    C. First changes are usually prolongation of cortical transit time, seen as cortical retention on scintigrams.
    D. Decreased EI.
    E. Severe rejection can cause no flow or function, or even a photopenic area.
IV. Chronic rejection.
    A. Decreased flow.
    B. Decreased function.
    C. Long-standing—chronic rejection may occasionally lead to renal tubular acidosis. Condition characterized by diminished renal perfusion and accumulation of OIH with near normal serum creatinine level.
V. Cyclosporine toxicity.
    A. Frequently preserved flow.
    B. Decreased function.
VI. Renal artery stenosis.
    A. Usually occurs after first month.
    B. Often has very slow insidious onset.
    C. Findings—similar to those of native kidneys.
    D. Normal EI.
    E. Upright position may promote prolongation of transit time.
VII. Urinoma.
    A. Findings.
  1. A photopenic area is seen on early images that fills on delayed images (up to 2 to 4 hours later).
VIII. Lymphocele.
    A. Photopenic region that does not fill in with time.
IX. Hematoma.
    A. Findings similar to lymphocele.
X. Urinary extravasation.
    A. Appearance of radionuclide outside confines of genitourinary (GU) tract. Technetium superior to hippuran for delineation.
    B. Urine leaks usually occur near ureterovesicular junction where an anastomosis of transplanted ureter into bladder wall may be complicated by:
      1. Ischemic necrosis.
      2. Rejection.
      3. Transient obstruction.

XI. Obstruction.
  A. May occur due to scar formation at site of anastomosis, blood clots, calculi, or extrinsic pressure caused by lymphocele, hematoma, or abscess.
  B. Findings similar to obstruction in a native kidney.
  C. With decreased function, delayed imaging may be necessary to appreciate obstruction.
XII. Subsegmental renal infarction.
  A. May occur in normal transplant or as consequence of chronic rejection.
  B. May be associated with hypertension.
  C. Presents as focal defect on function views.

Additional Radiopharmaceuticals

I. Other radiopharmaceuticals used to diagnose rejection.
  A. Technetium 99m sulfur colloid.
    1. Colloid is entrapped in fibrin network and deposited in glomerular arterioles and in area of vasculitis associated with endothelial proliferation.
    2. Findings.
      a. Increased sulfur colloid in comparison to adjacent bony structures.
    3. False-negative results.
      a. Anticoagulants.
      b. Nonfunctioning kidney.
      c. More than 14 days after transplantation (chronic).
    4. False-positive results.
      a. Normals.
      b. ATN.
      c. Infection.
      d. High-dose steroids.
  B. Labeled fibrinogen.
    1. Uptake in forming radioactive thrombi.
    2. Positive result—kidney/heart ratio greater than 1.2.
    3. False-negatives.
      a. Anticoagulants.
      b. Nonfunctioning kidneys.
    4. False-positives.
      a. Wound infection.
      b. Hematoma.
      c. Urinary leak.
      d. Infection.
  C. Gallium 67.

1. Uptake observed as normal finding during immediate postoperative period.
2. False-negatives.
   a. Necrotic acutely rejecting kidneys.
   b. Chronic rejection.
   c. Anticoagulants.
3. False-positives.
   a. Immediately postoperative period as noted above.
   b. ATN.
D. Indium 111 platelets.
   1. Increased deposition in acute rejection.
   2. False-negatives in chronic rejection.

VESICOURETERAL REFLUX

I. Background.
   A. Normal valve action at ureterovesicular junction depends on:
      1. Oblique entry of ureter into bladder.
      2. Adequate length of intramural ureter.
      3. Contraction of ureterotrigonal muscles.
      4. Active ureteral peristalsis.
   B. Reflux is associated with urinary tract infections (UTIs). Approximately 50% of those with UTIs in first year have reflux. Decreases as child grows older.
   C. Reflux usually resolves spontaneously by puberty; however, most critical period for development of reflux nephropathy is infancy and early childhood.
   D. Reflux of low grade more likely to spontaneously· disappear than those with high-grade reflux.
II. Technique.
   A. Have patient void.
   B. Catheterize patient.
   C. Fill bladder to capacity using bottle with hydrostratic pressure 70 to 90 cm water; this should contain 1 mCi of technetium.
   D. Multiple sequential images should be obtained during filling process; when capacity reached, patient should void.
   E. In some institutions, catheter is pulled; patient sits upright and voids into bedpan. In other institutions, patient voids with catheter in place.
   F. Imaging continues during voiding and postvoiding phase.
   G. Changing counts over bladder are compared with urine volume to calculate conversion factor; this allows quantitation of degree of reflux in milliliters with attenuation correction

$$\frac{\text{bladder counts}}{\text{urine vol}} = \text{correction factor}$$

H. Findings.
   1. In virtually 100% of patients in whom reflux occurs, it does so during micturition. Those showing reflux during both filling and micturition, 80%; micturition only, 20%.
   2. Reflux usually increases as study progresses; however, reflux can occasionally be transient.
   3. Note: There usually is a threshold volume under which reflux will not occur. When following patients serially, this threshold volume will increase during filling phase, indicating maturation of the ureterovesical junction.
   4. In phantom studies, can detect as small as 0.25-ml reflux.
   5. Can quantitate degree of reflux within 10% error.
   6. Grading system.
      a. Mild (grades 1 to 2 radiographically)—activity confined to ureter, especially distal ureter.
      b. Moderate (grade 3)—activity extends to pelvicalyceal system.
      c. Severe (grades 4 to 5)—distended redundant collecting system.

III. Advantages over radiographic voiding cystourethrogram (VUR).
   A. Radiation exposure of VUR very low.
      1. Bladder wall—18 to 27 mrad.
      2. Ovary—1 to 2 mrad.
      3. Testicle—even lower than in ovary.
      4. Radiographic techniques—50 to 200 times greater radiation exposure.

IV. Other techniques:
   A. Indirect method.
      1. Renal scanning agents such as DTPA or hippuran are injected IV. Patient is asked to void 1 to 2 hours later when most of tracer has cleared the upper tract and is in bladder.

TESTICULAR SCANNING

I. Anatomy (Fig. 6-1).
   A. Scrotum—cutaneous pouch that contains testes and parts of spermatic cord. The layers are skin and tunica dartos, which is a highly vascular, thin layer of fibrous tissue containing elastic and smooth-muscle fibers.
   B. Testis—covered by tunica albuginea, which is composed of dense, fibrous connective tissue.

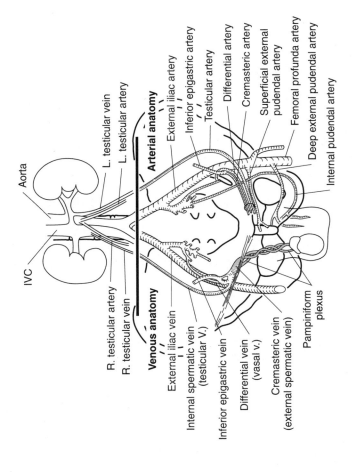

Fig. 6-1   Blood supply to testes and associated structures.

    C. Epididymis—comma-shaped structure lying on posterolateral surface of testis.

    D. Spermatic cord—fascia-covered cord containing blood vessels, lymph vessels, and nerves. Suspends testicle in scrotum. Affords involuntary testicular movement with cremasteric muscle.

    E. Tunica vaginalis—invaginated serous sac that covers testis, epididymis, and lower end of spermatic cord. Reflects onto itself to leave posterior border of the testis uncovered. This is area through which blood vessels and nerves enter testis via spermatic cord.

    F. Appendix testis—remnant of müllerian duct (paramesonephric), which regresses cranially.

    G. Appendix of epididymis—remnant of wolffian duct (mesonephric). May persist at cranial portion of testis.

    H. Paradidymis—paragenital tubules may persist.

II. Vascular supply.

    A. Testes—arterial supply (see Fig. 6-1).

        1. Testicular artery—provides principal blood supply for testis and epididymis. Originates from abdominal aorta just below renal artery. Joins spermatic cord above internal inguinal ring.

        2. Deferential artery—supplies the vas deferens. Anastomosis with testicular artery. Originates from hypogastric or vesicular arteries.

        3. Cremasteric artery—least important. Originates from inferior epigastric at level of inguinal ring. Like others, is part of spermatic cord.

    B. Testes—venous supply.

        1. Pampiniform plexus—consists of three freely anastomosing groups of veins.

        2. Testicular vein.

            a. Right—empties into inferior vena cava.

            b. Left—drains into renal vein. It is thought that acute angle of drainage into inferior vena cava sets stage for blockade of venous drainage, resulting in varicocele.

        3. Deferential vein.

        4. Cremasteric vein.

    C. Scrotum—arterial supply.

        1. Does not travel through spermatic cord. Does not anastomose with vessels supplying the testes, therefore cannot support testicular viability.

            a. Internal pudendal artery.

      b. Superficial pudendal artery.

      c. External pudendal artery.

III. Embryology.

  A. Testes migrate from abdomen to scrotum. A peritoneal out-pouching, the processus vaginalis accompanies it. Reflected fold of processus vaginalis becomes tunica vaginalis.

  B. Failure of testicular descent or anchorage results in ectopic location. Ectopic locations have higher incidence of torsion. Location of ectopic testis:

    1. Inguinal canal.

    2. Femoral canal.

    3. Suprapubic area.

IV. Pathophysiology.

  A. Normally tunica vaginalis covers only testis and anterolateral portion of epididymis. This allows posterior aspect of epididymis to attach to scrotal wall via connective tissue. Anchoring prevents torsion.

  B. Torsion can occur when complete envelopment of testis, epididymis, and distal spermatic cord by tunica vaginalis occurs (Fig. 6-2). Distal spermatic cord, testis, and epididymis are freely suspended within two layers of tunica vaginalis and, like clapper of a bell, are free to swing within the mobile environment. Abnormality termed "bell clapper deformity."

  C. Twisting of testicle causes veins to obstruct because of thin, easily compressed walls. The swollen veins can produce sufficient pressure to shut off arterial flow, even if twist itself has failed to occlude the artery. Loss of vascular supply leads to edema and congestion of compromised testicle, which is then followed by hemorrhage, and finally infarction.

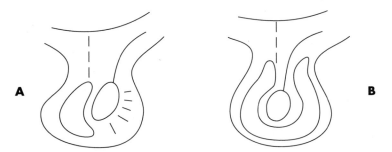

Fig. 6-2 Normally, **A**, testes are tethered posteriorly. In abnormal situations, **B**, tunica vaginalis envelopes testes, forming a "bell clapper" deformity.

V. Clinical findings.
  A. Torsion.
    1. Incidence—1 in 4,000 males at risk.
    2. Age—peak age, 14 years. May occur in utero. Rare after 30 years of age.
    3. Frequent onset during sleep. May be related to high testosterone level or relaxation.
    4. Pain—acute onset. Usually localized to scrotum. May elicit history of previous episodes that resolved spontaneously (spontaneous detorsion). May have low-grade fever. May be accompanied by nausea and vomiting. Usually *no* urinary symptoms. If an undescended testicle, may have abdominal pain.
    5. Laboratory results—urinalysis normal.
    6. Physical examination findings.
      a. Swollen, tender testicle.
      b. Detection of transverse lie on unaffected side with patient standing—indicates "bell clapper" deformity present. It is frequently bilateral.
  B. Epididymitis.
    1. Incidence—most common disease involving scrotum or contents.
    2. Age—usually in adult population. Below 14 years of age, very uncommon.
    3. Four varieties.
      a. Nonspecific epididymitis—most common variety. Misnomer, usually sequelae of infected urine. Common organisms: *Staphylococcus,* colon bacilli, *Streptococcus.* Reach epididymis by retrograde migration through the vas from established sites of infection in urine, posterior urethra, prostate, or seminal vesicles. May also spread by retrograde lymphatic pathways.
      b. Specific epididymitis—caused by gonorrhea; 25% of patients with gonococcal urethritis develop epididymitis. Also seen in second stage of syphilis, tuberculosis, etc.
      c. Traumatic epididymitis—may be a result of trauma itself or trauma may activate a dormant infection. May allow saprophytic organisms normally present in posterior urethra to gain access to epididymis.
      d. Mumps epididymo-orchitis—occurs in older boys or men. No prior history of mumps. There *may or may not be* preceding or concomitant episode of parotitis, since in adolescents and adults, mumps may initially manifest itself as epididymo-orchitis.

4. Physical examination—tender enlargement of epididymis situated posterolaterally, capping the testis. Often difficult to appreciate in patient with significant inflammation. Fever, prostatic tenderness common.
5. Laboratory results.
   a. Leukocytosis.
   b. Pyuria.
C. Torsion of appendix testis, appendix epididymis, or paradidymis—can mimic testicular torsion but not clinically important.
D. Hydrocele—collection of fluid between layers of tunica vaginalis.
   1. Primary hydrocele results from defect in lymphatic drainage, with accumulation of fluid.
   2. Secondary hydroceles associated with inflammatory disease, trauma, testicular tumor, etc.
E. Varicocele—abnormal dilatation and tortuosity of veins of pampiniform plexus within scrotum because of incompetency of valves permitting retrograde passage of blood; 99% left-sided resulting from:
   1. Right-angle termination left renal vein leading to obstruction.
   2. Compression of left renal vein between aorta and superior mesenteric artery.
   3. Presence of adrenalin-laden blood in left renal vein.
F. Inguinal hernia—prolapse of intraabdominal contents, most often intestine, into a patent processus vaginalis. Processus patent in almost all newborns; 60%, 1-year-olds; 20%, adult males. Hernia is 10 times more common in boys than men, presumably due to larger processus. Occur more often on right than left side, 10% bilateral.
G. Testicular tumors—most common neoplasms in men age 20 to 35. Tumors most often of germ-cell origin.
   1. Seminoma.
   2. Embryonal carcinoma.
   3. Teratoma.
   4. Choriocarcinoma.
VI. Scanning technique.
A. Administer 0.4 to 1 g of potassium perchlorate orally to block thyroid uptake of free pertechnetate.
B. Penis is taped up over pubis.
C. A tape sling or towel support is arranged to hold scrotum. Important that swollen testicle does not overlap normal testicle.
D. Scrotum placed in center of field.

E. A standard-field-of-view camera best. If large-field-of-view camera used, attempt to use magnifying capabilities. Converging collimator best. Parallel-hole collimator acceptable. In pediatric cases, pinhole collimator necessary on delayed views.

F. Initial set of images performed without lead shield. Lead shield then placed and re-imaged.

G. Fifteen to 20 mCi pertechnetate injected as a bolus in antecubital fossa. Minimum dose, 2 to 5 mCi.

H. Flow study performed using 3- to 6-second frames for approximately 60 seconds.

I. Several sets of "delayed" images begun immediately after flow study. Acquire for approximately 700,000 counts.

J. It is important to correlate physical location of testes with scan findings. This is done by physical examination and placing markers.

VII. Radionuclide findings.

A. Normal.

1. Flow study—medial border of iliac artery is smooth. No significant activity is seen in area of testicular, deferential, or pudendal artery. Scrotal perfusion, if present at all, is seen only as poorly marginated, minimally intense area of activity.

2. Tissue phase—scrotum and contents blur into homogeneous area of activity similar in intensity to the thigh. Dartos activity difficult to separate from epididymal or testicular activity. Better separated with lead shielding.

B. Torsion—depends on length of symptoms.

1. Acute—several hours after onset of symptoms.

a. Perfusion scan—normal or absent perfusion to affected side.

b. Tissue phase—photopenic area with activity less than opposite testicle and less than that of thigh. Increased activity may be seen high in cord, perhaps because of pooling in veins of pampiniform plexus or cut off of arterial flow in this region.

2. Missed torsion—delayed diagnosis resulting in infarction.

a. Perfusion scan—hyperemia through pudendal vessels. Adjacent inflammation causes Dartos hyperemia.

b. Tissue phase—bull's-eye or halo sign with surrounding rim of increased activity and central lucency. Central lucency usually, but not always, has less activity than opposite testicle or thigh.

3. Spontaneous detorsion.

a. Perfusion scan—increased flow.

b. Tissue phase—increased activity. Note that this may be difficult to differentiate from epididymitis (see below).

4. Torsion of appendages—indistinguishable from inflammatory disease. Evidence of epididymitis on scan in young patient with normal urinalysis—torsion of appendages.

C. Epididymitis.

1. Acute epididymitis.

a. Flow study—increased flow through spermatic cord vessels. Curvilinear laterally placed increased activity corresponding to posterolateral location of inflamed epididymis.

b. Tissue phase—increased activity.

c. Variations.

(1) Often, epididymis displaced medially, resulting in medially placed linear or curvilinear increased activity in scrotum on perfusion and tissue phases.

(2) If epididymal infection more focal (confined to head, body, or tail) flow study may not demonstrate abnormal increased flow through cord vessels, but only focal increase of tracer in scrotum. Tissue phase again shows only tiny spot of increased tracer. Should not be confused with torsion because there is no photopenic cool central region.

2. Acute epididymal orchitis.

a. Similar to acute epididymitis, but more medial testicular involvement seen.

D. Abscess—findings similar to missed torsion. Increased flow with halo/bull's-eye sign.

E. Hydrocele—appears as photopenic area in scrotal skin. Can be confused with a torsion. Transillumination/palpation helpful. May see hotter testicle in center of cooler hydrocele.

F. Varicocele—when of sufficient size, angiogram shows venous-phase accumulation that is also present on tissue phase.

G. Inguinal hernia.

1. Perfusion study—normal.

2. Tissue phase—photopenic area extending from inguinal region to hemiscrotum.

H. Scrotal trauma.

1. Flow study—diffusely increased.

2. Tissue phase—diffuse increase with decreased areas (due to hematoma, hematocele, hydrocele).

I. Tumor—findings variable.

1. Flow study—diffuse increased uptake.

2. Tissue phase—diffuse increased with decreased areas.
VIII. Utility of scan for torsion/epididymitis.
    A. Sensitivity—96%.
    B. Specificity—98%.
    C. Accuracy—96%.

SUGGESTED READINGS

Ash JM, Antico VF, Gilday DL, et al: Special considerations in the pediatric use of radionuclides for kidney studies. *Semin Nucl Med* 1982; 12:345-369.

Berg BC: Nuclear medicine and complementary modalities in renal trauma. *Semin Nucl Med* 1982; 12:280-303.

Chen DCP, Holder LE, Melloul M: Radionuclide scrotal imaging: Further experience with 210 new patients. I. Anatomy, pathophysiology, and methods. *J Nucl Med* 1983; 24:735-742.

Chen DCP, Holder LE, Melloul M: Radionuclide scrotal imaging: Further experience with 210 new patients. II. Results and discussion. *J Nucl Med* 1983; 24:841-853.

Conway JJ: "Well-tempered" diuresis renography: Its historical development, physiological and technical pitfalls, and standardized technique protocol. *Semin Nucl Med* 1992; 22:74-84.

Conway JJ, Kruglik GD: Effectiveness of direct and indirect radionuclide cystography in detecting vesicoureteral reflux. *J Nucl Med* 1975; 17:81-83.

Dubofsky EV, Russell CD: Quantitation of renal function with glomerular and tubular agents. *Semin Nucl Med* 1982; 12:308-329.

Eshima D, Taylor A: Technetium-99m (^{99m}Tc) mercaptoacetyltriglycine: Update on the new ^{99m}Tc renal tubular function agent. *Semin Nucl Med* 1992; 22:61-73.

Fine EJ: Interventions in renal scintirenography. *Semin Nucl Med* 1991; 21:116-127.

Fine EJ, Scharf SC, Blaufox MD: The role of nuclear medicine in evaluating the hypertensive patient. In Freeman LM, Weissmann HS (eds): *Nuclear medicine annual, 1984.* New York, Raven, 1984, pp 23-79.

Gates GF: Computation of glomerular filtration rate with Tc-99m DTPA: An in-house computer program. *J Nucl Med* 1984; 25:613-618.

Gates GF: Split renal function testing using Tc-99m DTPA: A rapid technique for determining glomerular filtration. *Clin Nucl Med* 1983; 8:400-407.

George EA: Radionuclide diagnosis of allograft rejection. *Semin Nucl Med* 1982; 12:379-386.

Gruenewald SM, Collins LT: Renovascular hypertension: Quantitative renography as a screening test. *Radiology* 1983; 140:287-291.

Handmaker H: Nuclear renal imaging in acute pyelonephritis. *Semin Nucl Med* 1982; 12:246-253.

Holder LE, Melloul M, Chen D: Current status of radionuclide scrotal imaging. *Semin Nucl Med* 1981; 11:232-249.

Kim EE, Pjura G, Lowry P, et al: Cyclosporin-A nephrotoxicity and acute cellular rejection in renal transplant recipients: Correlation between radionuclide and histologic findings. *Radiology* 1986; 159:443-446.

Kirchner PT, Rosenthall L: Renal transplant evaluation. *Semin Nucl Med* 1982; 12:370-378.

Krueter RP, Ash JM, Silver MM, et al: Primary hydronephrosis: Assessment of diuretic renography, pelvis perfusion pressure, operative findings, and renal and ureteral histology. *Urol Clin North Am* 1980; 7:231-242.

Leonard JC, Allen EW, Goin J, et al: Renal cortical imaging and the detection of renal mass lesions. *J Nucl Med* 1979; 20:1018-1022.

Lutzker LG: The fine points of scrotal scintigraphy. *Semin Nucl Med* 1982; 12:387-393.

Mann SJ, Pickering TG: Detection of renovascular hypertension: State of the art. *Ann Int Med* 1992; 117:845-853.

Nally JV, Black HR: State-of-the-art review: Captopril renography: Pathophysiological considerations and clinical observations. *Semin Nucl Med* 1992; 22:85-97.

Powers TA, Stone WJ, Grove B, et al: Radionuclide measurement of differential glomerular filtration rate. *Invest Radiol* 1981; 16:59-64.

Scharf SC, Blaufox MD: Radionuclides in the evaluation of urinary obstruction. *Semin Nucl Med* 1982; 12:254-264.

Sfakianakis GN, Bourgoignie JJ, Jaffe D, et al: Single-dose captopril scintigraphy in the diagnosis of renovascular hypertension. *J Nucl Med* 1987; 28:1383-1392.

Tanaka T, Mishkin F, Datta NS: Radionuclide imaging of the scrotal contents. In Freeman LM, Weissman HS (eds): *Nuclear medicine annual, 1981*. New York, Raven, 1981, pp 195-222.

Taylor AT: Quantitation of renal function with static imaging agents. *Semin Nucl Med* 1982; 12:330-344.

Taylor AT: Quantitative renal function scanning: A historical and current status report on renal radiopharmaceuticals. In Freeman LM, Weissmann HS (eds): *Nuclear medicine annual, 1980*. New York, Raven, 1980, pp 303-340.

Tauxe WN, Dubovsky EV, Kidd T, et al: New formulas for the calculation of effective renal plasma flow. *Eur J Nucl Med* 1982; 7:51-54.

Thrall JH, Koff SA, Keyes JW: Diuretic radionuclide renography and scintigraphy in the differential diagnosis of hydroureteronephrosis. *Semin Nucl Med* 1981; 11:89-104.

7

Cardiac Imaging

HEART
Anatomy

I. Blood supply.
  A. Left coronary artery—3 main branches:
    1. Left anterior descending—supplies:
       a. Anterolateral wall of left ventricle (LV).
       b. Interventricular septum anteriorly.
    2. Left circumflex—supplies:
       a. Posterolateral wall of left ventricle.
       b. Left atrium.
    3. Obtuse marginal branches.
  B. Right coronary artery.
    1. Posterior descending artery.
    2. In 80% of people, right coronary is dominant—i.e., is origin of posterior descending artery.
    3. Supplies:
       a. Inferior wall of left ventricle.
       b. Variable portion of interventricular septum.
       c. Right ventricle.
       d. Right atrium.

Physiology

I. Contraction.
  A. Wall motion.
    1. Left ventricle.
       a. Greatest movement is anterior wall. Left ventricle normally shortens 40% along short axis.
       b. Apex moves significantly less; long axis normally shortens approximately 20%.
       c. Least movement seen in septum; thickens slightly and moves medially minimal amount; movement greater for lower septum near apex than for basilar portion.
       d. Wall motion often graded as:

        (1) 3+ = normal.

        (2) 2+ = mild hypokinesis.

        (3) 1+ = severe hypokinesis.

        (4) 0 = akinesis.

        (5) −1 = dyskinesis; indicates wall moves outward during ventricular systole.

    2. Right ventricle.

      a. Three main movements of right ventricular wall cause ejection of blood:

        (1) Apex moves upward.

        (2) Tricuspid valve plane moves downward.

        (3) Septum thickens.

II. Ejection fraction (EF) and other parameters.

  A. Left ventricle.

    1. End-diastolic volume (EDV)—amount of blood in left ventricle at end diastole.

      a. Normal—150 ml.

    2. Stroke volume—equals amount of blood ejected by ventricle during systole.

      a. Normal—80 to 100 ml.

    3. Cardiac output—volume of blood pumped by ventricle in 1 minute.

      a. Cardiac output = stroke volume × heart rate.

      b. Normal—5 to 6 L/minute.

    4. EF equals percentage of EDV pumped by ventricle per beat.

      a. $EF = \dfrac{\text{end diastolic volume} - \text{end systolic volume}}{\text{end diastolic volume}}$

      b. Normal—50% to 65%.

    5. EF is value used as indicator of overall cardiac function with gated blood pool study.

  B. Right ventricle.

    1. EDV = 165 ml.

    2. EF = 45% to 60%.

    3. Because stroke volumes must be equal on left and right side of heart and because right ventricular EDV is larger than left, RV EF must be lower than LV.

    4. Note that if gated first-pass technique used to determine right ventricular EF, *due to the technique, normal values are actually higher for the right than the left ventricle.* However, numbers are *proportional* to true right ventricular EF.

III. Coronary blood flow.

  A. Myocardial blood flow greatest during diastole. Coronary vessels

are not being constricted by contraction of cardiac muscle at this time.
B. With exercise, coronary blood flow increases threefold to sixfold.
C. With narrowing of coronary vessel less than 50% of diameter, effect on blood flow is relatively insignificant.
D. As narrowing approaches 70%, lesion hemodynamically significant *during exercise*. Resting coronary flow not greatly reduced until stenosis greater than 85%. Thus, exercise studies are used to diagnose coronary ischemic disease.

Radiopharmaceuticals

I. Thallium 201.
  A. Physical characteristics.
    1. Cyclotron-produced. Impure, contains lead 203 and thallium 202.
    2. Decays by electron capture.
    3. Mercury 201 emits mercury K characteristic x-rays of 69 to 83 keV. This is main energy emitted. In addition, gamma rays with low abundance also emitted at 167 keV (10%) and 135 keV (3%). Some institutions image these photons, as well, to improve photon flux.
    4. Physical half-life—73 hours.
  B. Biokinetics.
    1. Group IIIA metal.
    2. Biologic properties similar, but not identical to, potassium. Ionic radii both elements extremely similar. Distribution of thallium ions following IV administration primarily intracellular, like potassium.
    3. Thallium transport across cell membrane dependent on sodium potassium pump (controversial).
  C. Initial distribution.
    1. Initial regional myocardial concentration of thallium is dependent on:
      a. Regional blood flow.
        (1) Main determinant.
        (2) Regional myocardial uptake of thallium is *proportional* to blood flow. As coronary blood flow increases above baseline level, myocardial uptake of thallium increases. Similarly, as regional myocardial blood flow falls, thallium uptake falls.
      b. Extraction fraction.
        (1) Normally 85% of thallium in coronary blood removed by myocardium in single pass.
        (2) Extraction fraction *not* affected by:

(a) Acidosis.
(b) Beta-adrenergic blockers.
(c) Insulin.
(d) Digitalis.

(3) Extraction fraction *decreases with:*
(a) Extremely high coronary blood flow rates.
(i) Exercise.
(ii) Vasodilators.

2. Because 5% of cardiac output flows through coronary arteries and extraction efficiency equals 85%, approximately 4% of total injected dose is localized in heart.

3. Five percent to 15% injected dose extracted by lungs before reaching systemic circulation.
a. If pulmonary circulation time is slow, amount taken up is higher. Thus, patients with left ventricular failure will have lower heart-to-lung uptake ratios.

4. Initial myocardial uptake of thallium rapid—peak approximately 10 minutes.

5. Remaining approximately 90% distributes into other body organs. Those with highest uptake include:
(1) Skeletal muscle.
(2) Gastrointestinal tract.
(3) Kidneys—receive largest radiation dose-1.2 rad/mCi.

D. Redistribution.

1. Distribution of thallium in heart not static. Changes as a function of time. Change from initial myocardial ^{201}Tl distribution is called *redistribution.*

2. In patients in whom thallium injected during exercise, if ischemia present, initial perfusion defect seen. Delayed imaging shows disappearance of initial defect due to redistribution.

3. Disappearance of initial thallium defects over time is result of:
a. Accumulation of thallium in previously under-perfused zones.
b. Washout of radioactivity from normal myocardium.

4. Tissues in which initial uptake of thallium high in relation to potassium content lose thallium with time, while tissues with low initial uptake (ischemic but viable myocardium) gain activity.

5. Blood pool thallium continuously exchanges with myocardium as well as extracardiac organs.

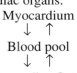

Myocardium
↓ ↑
Blood pool
↓ ↑
Extracardiac Organs

6. During redistribution, thallium both enters myocardium (from

systemic pool) and washes out of myocardium. The net difference between input and output is called *net myocardial washout rate*.

7. Local concentration of thallium continues to change until equilibrium condition is achieved, so ratio between input and output is constant.

8. Intrinsic washout rate (output) is monoexponential with $T\frac{1}{2}$ of approximately 1 hour. The net thallium washout rate (input and output) has a $T_{1/2}$ of 4 hours.

9. Washout rate depends primarily on initial deposition of thallium but can be increased by:
   a. Eating.
   b. Injection of glucose and insulin.

10. In reversible thallium defects, the *net* washout rate for thallium slower compared with normal areas. This is associated with viable myocardium.

11. In nonreversible defects, initial ratio of thallium concentration between normal and abnormal regions maintained over time because of similar net washout rates in normal and abnormal zones. This is associated with presence of myocardial scar. Note normal washout rates in region of scar may be secondary to normal washout in nonischemic areas superimposed on abnormal zone (with planar imaging).

II. ^{99m}Tc sestamibi (Sesta = 6; six methoxyisobutyl isonitrile [MIBI] ligands surround a technetium central core).

A. Physical characteristics.

1. Superior physical characteristics allow improved image quality over ^{201}Tl.
   a. 140 KeV photon of ^{99m}Tc is ideally suited to scintillation camera imaging.
   b. Half-value layer (thickness of soft tissue or water that attenuates 50% of photons) of ^{99m}Tc is 4.6 cm for ^{99m}Tc and only 3.7 for ^{201}Tl; thus, more photons are available for imaging.
   c. Physical half-life of 6 hours vs 73 hours for ^{201}Tl (plus the biodistribution of sestamibi vs ^{201}Tl) allows doses exceeding 30 mCi to be used while delivering radiation exposure $\leq$ 3.5 mCi of ^{201}Tl. Increased photon flux of ^{99m}Tc sestamibi is especially useful in SPECT imaging.

B. Dosimetry of ^{99m}Tc sestamibi vs ^{201}Tl at rest (Table 7-1).

C. Biokinetics.

1. Lipophilic cation enters myocardial cells via passive transport.
2. Binds to mitochondria.
3. Net accumulation dependent on normal mitochondrial func-

Table 7-1   Dosimetry of ^{201}Tl and ^{99m}Tc Sestamibi

	Dose (rads)	
	^{201}Tl (3.5 mCi)	^{99m}Tc Sestamibi (30 mCi)
Total body	0.7	0.5
Testes	1.8	0.4
Ovaries	1.6	2.0
Kidneys*	4.2	2.0
Upper large intestine†	0.9	5.4

*Critical organ for ^{201}Tl.
†Critical organ for ^{99m}Tc sestamibi.

tion. Net accumulation depressed and net washout increased during severe inhibition of aerobic cellular metabolism, such as during hypoxia secondary to severe ischemia.

D. Distribution.

1. Like ^{201}Tl, sestamibi is taken up by myocardium in proportion to bloodflow.
2. Cellular transport mechanism differs between the two agents.
   a. Peak extraction for sestamibi is approximately half that of ^{201}Tl.
3. Most significant difference from ^{201}Tl—sestamibi has almost no redistribution; therefore, it requires separate stress and rest injections.
4. Rest distribution.
   a. Highest initial concentration—gallbladder and liver (hepatobiliary system is major route of clearance—37%, followed by kidneys—25%).
   b. In descending order, heart, spleen and lungs have next highest concentration.
   c. Changes in activity with time.
      (1) Heart activity relatively stable.
      (2) Liver decreases with excretion into biliary system; gallbladder shows maximal activity at 60 minutes.
      (3) Splenic and lung activity decreases over time.
      (4) At 90 minutes, heart count density is greater than surrounding organs—adequate heart/background ratios for imaging by 60 to 90 minutes.
5. Stress distribution.
   a. Concentration, in descending order:
      (1) Gallbladder.
      (2) Heart.

  (3) Liver.
  (4) Spleen.
  (5) Lung.
 b. At all times after injection, cardiac activity is higher than immediately adjacent organs; therefore, imaging can commence earlier than after rest—30 to 60 minutes after injection.
III. ^{99m}Tc teboroxime—a BATO compound (boronic acid adducts of technetium dioxime complexes).
 A. Physical characteristics—same as sestamibi.
 B. Biokinetics.
  1. Lipophilic, chemically neutral agent that diffuses across phospholipid cell membrane.
  2. Has two to five times faster uptake and greater myocardial accumulation than sestamibi or thallium.
  3. Less sensitive to metabolic inhibition of uptake than sestamibi or ^{201}Tl; therefore, appealing as agent for determining myocardial viability.
  4. Greatest disadvantage—because of its neutral lipophilic properties, it is freely diffusable and has very rapid washout ($T_{1/2}$ 10 to 15 minutes), making imaging difficult.
   a. Triple-headed cameras best for obtaining rapid acquisition necessary.
  5. Kinetics of washout may be useful for diagnosing ischemia.
 C. Distribution.
  1. Liver is major organism of metabolism with uptake peaking at 6 minutes; excretion into bowel.

Technique

 I. Rest thallium study.
 A. Patient who has been given nothing by mouth for 4 to 6 hours is injected with 3 to 4 mCi ^{201}Tl IV.
 B. Patient should be in upright position for 15 minutes before injection, and during injection. This reduces pulmonary and splanchnic blood flow, decreasing background activity in these regions.
 C. Imaging instituted 20 minutes following injection. Delay is required because of slower blood clearance of thallium at rest.
 D. Planar imaging.
  1. Best to use gamma camera with 0.25-inch-thick crystal (rather than 0.50-inch-thick crystal) to improve resolution without significant loss in sensitivity.
  2. Best to use specially designed high-resolution parallel-square-hole collimator with thin septi. These offer high resolution

with higher relative sensitivity, compared to GAP collimators. Note that, because of thin septa, ^{201}Tl preparation must be used with small amounts of contaminating ^{202}Tl (439 keV), since these emissions go uncollimated, thereby degrading resolution. This limits the shelf-life of ^{201}Tl, since its physical half-life is 73 hours compared with 12 days for ^{202}Tl.

   3. If special collimator not available, general all-purpose parallel-hole collimator best compromise between sensitivity and resolution. High-resolution collimators not warranted in view of minimal improvement image quality for increased imaging time.

   4. A 20% window set is centered on 69 to 83 keV mercury photopeak. In systems with multiple pulse-height analyzers, may use 135- and 167-keV photopeaks as well.

   5. Acquire 500,000 counts/field. If cardiac shield used to remove liver activity, 300,000 counts sufficient.

   6. Anterior, left anterior oblique (LAO), and lateral views obtained.
     a. Left lateral view should be done in right decubitus position. This prevents diaphragmatic attenuation from causing apparent inferior defect in patients with normal inferior myocardial perfusion.

   7. "Redistribution" views may be obtained 3 to 4 hours later, even on resting. Redistribution of defects, even at rest, has been described. Thus, one can better differentiate scar from ischemia.

II. Stress study.
  A. Patient has nothing by mouth for 4 to 6 hours before examination.
  B. Patient placed on electrocardiographic (ECG) monitoring.
  C. An IV line is placed to allow easy injection during exercise.
  D. Graded treadmill exercise most commonly done, according to standard protocol such as Bruce protocol.
  E. Exercise carried out to patient's maximum heart rate.
  F. Test may be terminated early if any of the following occurs:
    1. Angina.
    2. Severe shortness of breath.
    3. Fall in blood pressure (BP).
    4. Ischemic ECG changes.
    5. Significant cardiac arrhythmias.
    6. Patient becomes exhausted.
    7. Patient reaches 85% of predicted maximum heart rate.
  G. Adequacy of exercise and resultant stress on myocardium may also be assessed by double product (heart rate × BP). This plus maximum heart rate correlates well with myocardial oxygen consumption.
  H. From 60 to 90 seconds before patient is to terminate exercise,

^{201}Tl is injected IV. During final exercise postinjection it is important that the patient maintain maximal stress and not slow down, so that distribution of thallium occurs at maximal stress.

I. Important that patient at least achieve 85% maximal exercise rates. Sensitivity may fall by as much as 50% with submaximal exercise.

J. Imaging performed as for rest study initially. Exception—initial imaging should begin at about 15 minutes after injection, to prevent problems from rapid redistribution.

K. Computer analysis of images sometimes performed with stress studies.

L. Patient should not eat heavily or exercise between initial and redistribution images.

M. Redistribution images are obtained at 4 hours after injection.

N. Alternative forms of stress.
   1. Bicycle ergometer.
      a. May be used instead of treadmill.
      b. Some patients unable to operate pedals; others experience early leg fatigue.
      c. Bicycle exercise in supine position produces lower maximal heart rate response.
   2. Isometric hand grip.
      a. Causes modest increase in BP without heart rate change, thus stress to myocardium not great. May increase alpha-adrenergic discharge to heart, which decreases size of coronary arteries and possibly initiates spasm.
   3. Cold pressor test.
      a. Immersion of hand in ice water.
      b. Physiology similar to hand grip.

III. Pharmacologic stress for myocardial perfusion imaging.
   A. Background.
      1. Myocardial perfusion scintigraphy.
         a. Uptake of ^{201}Tl and ^{99m}Tc sestamibi are proportional to regional blood flow.
         b. Differences in regional blood flow produce heterogeneity on scan.
         c. Heterogeneity is the primary finding used to diagnose CAD.
      2. Coronary artery disease.
         a. At rest, blood flow is normal through diseased vessels.
            (1) No regional differences in blood flow are present.
            (2) Scan is normal.
         b. With stress, diminished coronary flow reserve in diseased vessels.

       (1) Results in regional blood flow differences.

       (2) Scan shows cold defects.

3. Exercise stress.

   a. Produces increased myocardial oxygen consumption; this is reflected in increased double product.

   b. To supply increased needs, flow must increase through coronary vessels.

   c. Stenotic vessels (diminished flow reserve) cannot increase flow.

4. Pharmacologic stress agents.

   a. Dobutamine.

   b. Dipyridamole.

   c. Adenosine.

5. Pharmacologic stress produced by dobutamine.

   a. Similar to exercise.

   b. Indirectly tests flow reserve.

   c. Increases myocardial oxygen consumption.

       (1) Chronotropic effects.

       (2) Inotropic effects.

   d. Invokes ischemia; this results in cold defects on scan.

6. Pharmacologic stress using dipyridamole.

   a. Mechanism of action different from exercise.

   b. Directly tests flow reserve.

   c. Dipyridamole causes vasodilatation.

   d. Normal vessels vasodilate, increasing flow.

   e. Stenotic vessels are already maximally vasodilated, cannot increase flow.

   f. Results in heterogeneity on scan.

   g. Does not depend on induction of ischemia.

7. Adenosine.

   a. Action similar to that with dipyridamole.

8. Advantages of exercise stress.

   a. Electrocardiogram (ECG) information is more sensitive for ischemia than after pharmacologic stress.

   b. Prescribe exercise regimen after myocardial infarction (MI).

       (1) Can best determine the level of exercise allowed with stress test.

   c. Experience.

9. Disadvantages of exercise stress.

   a. Sensitivity for CAD depends on achieving maximal stress.

       (1) One third of patients "submax" on exercise studies.

       (2) Submaximal exercise reduces sensitivity of scan for ischemia by 50%.

      b. Some patients cannot exercise.

      c. Medications may limit level of stress.

        (1) Beta blockers.

        (2) Calcium channel blockers.

      d. Risk stratification not as accurate as with dipyridamole.

B. Clinical pharmacology.

  1. Dobutamine.

      a. Adrenergic agonist.

        (1) Chronotropic effects.

        (2) Ionotropic effects.

  2. Dipyridamole.

      a. Pyrimidine compound.

      b. Molecular weight 504.

      c. Lipophilic.

      d. Mildly acidic in solution.

      e. Mechanism of action.

        (1) Increases adenosine in blood.

        (2) Adenosine potent vasodilator.

        (3) Greatest effect on coronary vessels.

        (4) Inhibits uptake of adenosine by red blood cells and endothelium.

        (5) Also blocks inactivation of adenosine by adenosine deaminases.

      f. Increases coronary blood five times.

      g. In animals, 0.568 mg/kg over 4 minutes yields maximal coronary vasodilatation.

      h. Peak blood flow 6.5 minutes (2.5 to 8.7).

      i. Flow returns to baseline by 30 minutes.

      j. Heart rate (HR) increases 13 beats per minute (20%).

      k. Blood pressure (BP) decreases 6 mm Hg (2% to 8%).

      l. Metabolism and excretion.

        (1) Liver—converted to monoglucuronide.

        (2) Excreted in bile.

        (3) Hepatic dysfunction may enhance effects.

      m. Antidote—aminophylline. Blocks adenosine receptors.

C. Dipyridamole technique.

  1. Patient preparation.

      a. Nothing by mouth for minimum of 4 hours.

      b. Hold caffeine-containing materials for 24 to 36 hours.

        (1) Beverages—coffee, tea, and soft drinks.

        (2) Foods—chocolate.

        (3) Medications—stop preparations containing theophylline for 36 to 48 hours.

2. Drug preparation.
   a. Dilute at least 1:2 in 0.45%, 0.9% NaCl or in 5% D5W.
   b. Dilute to a total volume of 20 to 50 ml.
      (1) Allows convenient control of infusion rate.
      (2) Prevents local irritation.
3. Administration.
   a. Piggyback IV set or calibrated infusion pump.
   b. Dipyridamole dosage:
      (1) 0.142 mg/kg per minute over 4 minutes for total of 0.57 mg/kg.
      (2) Limit total dose to 60 mg.
4. Patient monitoring.
   a. Continuous ECG recording.
   b. Blood pressure and HR every 1 to 2 minutes; then as needed for next 30 minutes.
   c. Have aminophylline ready.
   d. Resuscitation equipment at bedside.
5. Thalium imaging procedure.
   a. Inject 2 to 5 minutes after the end of infusion.
   b. Image 10 minutes after injection of ^{201}Tl.
   c. Delayed imaging 3 to 4 hours later.
6. Sestamibi—use usual sestamibi protocol.
7. Addition of exercise—controversial.
   a. Further increases coronary blood flow.
   b. Reduces splanchnic blood flow.
   c. Types of exercise:
      (1) Isometric hand grip.
      (2) Bicycle pedaling against minimal resistance.
      (3) Low-level treadmill.
D. Adverse effects.
   1. Drug-related adverse events occur in 46.8% of patients.
   2. Drug-related mortality is 1 in 2000 (0.05%).
   3. Incidence of adverse reations to dipyridamole (%):
      a. Chest pain—19.7.
      b. ECG abnormalities—15.9.
      c. ST–T-wave changes only—7.5.
      d. Headache—12.2.
      e. Dizziness—11.8.
      f. Nausea or vomiting—5.0.
      g. Hypotension—4.6.
      h. Flushing or hot flashes—3.4.
      i. Dyspnea—2.6.
      j. Blood pressure lability—1.6.
      k. Hypertension—1.5.

l. Paresthesia—1.3.

m. Fatigue—1.2.

4. Chest pain .
    a. Infrequently due to ischemia.
    b. May be due to:
        (1) Esophageal spasm.
        (2) Adenosine-mediated stimulation of cardiac pain receptors.
5. ST-segment changes.
    a. Indicate ischemia.
        (1) Usually associated with an advanced, tight lesion.
6. Dipyridamole-induced ischemia.
    a. Coronary steal phenomenon.
    b. Reduced perfusion pressure.
7. Coronary steal phenomenon—shunting of augmented flow through normal vessels at expense of diseased vessels.
    a. May require specific anatomy to occur.
    b. Has been demonstrated in animals.
    c. Primarily affects subendocardium.
    d. PET studies have confirmed reduced flow in humans.
8. Reduced perfusion pressure.
    a. Occurs in face of full vasodilatation.
    b. Increase in the transstenotic gradient.
    c. Reduction in distal coronary perfusion pressure.
    d. Results in decreased subendocardial flow.
9. Serious adverse reactions reported in original study.
    a. Eight of 3,911 (0.2%).
    b. Two MIs.
    c. Six with severe bronchospasm.
10. Serious adverse reactions reported by others.
    a. Severe hypotension.
    b. Bradycardia and heart block.
11. Myocardial infarction.
    a. More common in patients with unstable angina.
    b. Especially likely if increasing anginal attack rate.
12. Bronchospasm.
    a. More common if patient has history of asthma or wheezing.
    b. Recent discontinuation of medications promotes bronchospasm.
13. Hypotension.
    a. More common if:
        (1) Blood pressure is unstable.
        (2) Resting systolic BP <100 mm Hg.

(3) Left ventricular function and HR response are depressed, such as post MI with pacemaker.
14. Adverse effects that should be treated include:
    a. Severe chest pain.
    b. ST-segment changes.
    c. Bronchospasm.
    d. Significant fall in BP.
    e. Severe headache.
    f. Nausea and vomiting.
E. Treatment of adverse reactions.
    1. Treatment—aminophylline.
        a. IV aminophylline dose 50 to 250 mg.
        b. Slow IV injection of 50 to 100 mg over 30 to 60 seconds.
        c. If chest pain persists—sublingual nitroglycerin.
        d. If possible, delay aminophylline 2 to 3 minutes after injection of ^{201}Tl; slightly longer for ^{99m}Tc sestamibi.
    2. Prophylactic aminophylline—controversial.
        a. Fifty to 100 mg 2 to 3 minutes after injection of ^{201}Tl.
        b. May prevent occurrence of side effects during imaging.
F. Diagnosis of CAD in 1,843 patients with dipyridamole.
    1. Sensitivity—86%.
    2. Similar to exercise.
G. Risk stratification.
    1. Preoperative risk.
        a. Peripheral vascular disease.
        b. Prerenal transplant.
    2. Preoperative risk following peripheral vascular surgery.
        a. MI is leading cause of perioperative and postoperative mortality.
        b. In one study:
            (1) Of patients who had abnormal dipyridamole ^{201}Tl scans preoperatively, 50% had perioperative cardiac events.
            (2) Of patients with normal dipyridamole scans, none had a perioperative event.
        c. In a second study:
            (1) Abnormal dipyridamole scan preoperatively—23 times greater risk of perioperative event.
            (2) Addition of ST-segment depression or history of diabetes—30 times greater risk.
    3. Post MI risk stratification.
        a. Abnormal dipyridamole scan:
            (1) Of patients readmitted for angina, 92% had abnormal scans.

   (2) Of those with recurrent MI or death, 92% had abnormal scans.

   (3) Only factor associated with occurrence of cardiac events.

H. Adenosine.

 1. Naturally occurring nucleotide.

 2. Mediators of energy metabolism—cyclic AMP and ATP.

 3. Potent vasodilator.

 4. Adenosine versus dipyridamole.

  a. Adenosine direct action.

  b. Dipyridamole indirect.

  c. Increases adenosine.

 5. Mode of action.

  a. Adenosine interacts with adenosine A_2 receptors. ,

  b. Increases adenyl cyclase and cyclic AMP.

  c. Decreases sarcolemic calcium uptake.

  d. Leads to vasodilatation.

 6. Clinical pharmacology.

  a. Increases blood flow four to five times above baseline.

  b. Maximal coronary flow increase at 140 µg/kg per minute.

  c. Ultrashort half-life of 2 to 10 seconds.

 7. Antidote.

  a. Turning off infusion.

  b. Aminophylline rarely needed.

 8. Metabolism and excretion.

  a. Returns to intracellular space and is metabolized to uric acid.

  b. Regenerates ATP and SAM.

 9. Physiologic effects.

  a. Increase of HR by 10 beats per minute.

  b. Reduction in BP by 10 mm Hg.

 10. Adenosine technique.

  a. Patient preparation—same as with dipyridamole.

  b. Drug administration.

   (1) Pump infusion.

   (2) Drug dosage—140 µg/kg for 6 minutes.

  c. Imaging technique.

   (1) Inject ^{201}Tl at 3 minutes.

   (2) Continue adenosine infusion for 3 more minutes.

   (3) Begin imaging 11 minutes after start of infusion.

   (4) Delayed imaging at 4 hours.

 11. Drug adverse effects—adenosine versus dipyridamole.

  a. Significantly higher with adenosine than with dipyridamole.

    b. Observed drug adverse effects (%):

      (1) Chest pain—51.

      (2) ECG changes—12.

      (3) Headache—35.

      (4) Facial flushing—29.

      (5) Shortness of breath—15.

      (6) First-degree atrioventricular (AV) block—10.

      (7) Second-degree AV block—2.

      (8) Third-degree AV block—0.5.

    c. Atrioventricular block:

      (1) Adenosine inhibits AV node conduction.

        (a) Used to treat supraventricular tachycardias.

      (2) Tends to start in first 1 to 2 minutes of infusion.

      (3) Almost always transient, lasting a few beats.

      (4) Has not caused symptoms of diminished systemic or cerebral perfusion.

    d. High-risk patients include those with:

      (1) Unstable angina.

      (2) Recent MI.

      (3) Hypotension.

      (4) Bronchospasm.

    e. Patients who should not be studied include those with:

      (1) Sick sinus syndrome.

      (2) Second- or third-degree AV block. Note: First-degree AV block and bundle branch block have no increased risk.

      (3) Hypotension at rest (systolic BP <80 mm Hg).

12. Technique for high-risk patients.

    a. Infuse at initial rate of 50 μg/kg per minute.

    b. Observe for side effects.

    c. Increase dose at 1-minute intervals—50 to 75 to 100 to 140 μg/kg per minute.

    d. Inject ^{201}Tl at 3 minutes.

    e. Continue infusion at maximal rate for 3 more minutes.

13. Treatment of adverse effects.

    a. Reduce infusion rate to tolerable level.

      (1) 75 to 100 μg/kg per minute.

        (a) Still increases coronary blood flow two to four times.

    b. Continue infusion for minimum of 1 minute after ^{201}Tl injection.

14. Sensitivity and specificity for CAD.

    a. Sensitivity—86%.

    b. Specificity—90%.

IV. Single-photon emission computed tomography (SPECT).
  A. Protocol above modified as follows:
    1. Quality control *very* important.
      a. Flood correction matrix for uniformity correction.
        (1) Needs to be performed, to correct for variations in PM tube and collimator performance.
        (2) With round camera, 30 million count extrinsic flood (for 64 × 64 matrix) or 120 million count (for 128 × 128 matrix) done weekly.
        (3) With a square or rectangular camera, 40 million count extrinsic flood (64 × 64 matrix) or 160 million count flood done weekly.
      b. Center-of-rotation correction (COR).
        (1) Center-of-rotation can "drift." COR is performed to correct electromechanical misalignment so that physical center of camera corresponds to electronic matrix center.
        (2) Performed weekly.
      c. As with any camera, perform daily flood of 2.5 million counts and weekly bar phantom as checks of system performance.
    2. Set up camera as follows:
      a. 64 × 64 image matrix with a hardware zoom of 1.3 to 1.5.
      b. 180° arc from left posterior oblique (LPO) 45° to right anterior oblique (RAO) 45°.
      c. 32 to 64 stops with total acquisition time of 30 minutes.
      d. Reconstruction and filtering are system dependent.
    3. Inject 3.5 mCi of ^{201}Tl and continue stress (or do not reverse pharmacologic stress) for at least 60 seconds.
    4. Wait 15 minutes before imaging to prevent heart creep. As noted in computer-assisted diagnosis section: Immediately after exercise, deep breathing depresses diaphragm and heart. As patients catch their breath, heart and diaphragm creep up, which can produce artifactual defects in inferoposterior wall. Waiting 15 minutes allows patient to return to quiet breathing before initiating imaging.
    5. While waiting, perform 300,000-count anterior planar image over chest to evaluate for pulmonary uptake. Place a region-of-interest over areas of left lung and myocardium with highest activity. Mean counts per pixel in lung are divided by those in myocardial region of interest. Values above 0.3 to 0.5 are abnormal; however, each laboratory must establish its own criteria.
      a. Increased uptake is a marker of coronary artery disease (CAD) and often indicates multivessel disease.

      b. Mechanism is related to increased pulmonary hypertension and slow transit.

    6. Perform delayed imaging 4 hours later.

      a. Before imaging, inject 1 mCi of ^{201}Tl to better determine reversibility (see viability discussion).

V. ^{99m}Tc sestamibi imaging protocols.

  A. One-day stress-rest protocol.

    1. Patient is placed NPO past midnight.

    2. Rest study is performed.

      a. Patient is injected with 8 to 9 mCi sestamibi.

      b. Eight ounces of whole milk or light fatty meal is ingested between injection and imaging (some give it halfway between injection and imaging; others give it as late as 15 minutes before imaging). Fatty meal causes gallbladder contraction, reducing the radioactivity in it.

      c. Imaging performed 60 to 90 minutes after injection.

    3. At 0 to 4 hours (best to wait 3 to 4 hours) exercise study is performed. Time delay of 3 to 4 hours allows 29% to 37% of rest dose to decay, reducing background activity.

      a. Patient is injected with 22 to 25 mCi at peak exercise or pharmacologic stress. Exercise is continued at least 1 minute after sestamibi injection (with dipyridamole stress, best not to reverse, or at least wait 1 to 4 minutes after injection).

      b. Milk is given again.

      c. Imaging is begun 30 to 60 minutes after injection.

    4. Although stress can be performed first, studies indicate this protocol yields poorer differentiation of ischemia from scars.

  B. Two-day protocol.

    1. Similar to one-day protocol, *except:*

      a. Exercise performed day 1.

      b. Rest performed day 2.

      c. For each study 22 mCi used.

  C. Planar imaging.

    1. Place patient in supine position.

    2. Use large-field-of-view (LFOV) camera with general all-purpose or high-resolution collimator.

    3. Twenty percent windows centered on 140 KeV with 1.2 to 1.5 zoom and 128 × 128 matrix.

    4. At least 1 million counts per image—about 5 to 8 minutes per view.

    5. Obtain anterior 45-degree LAO and 70-degree LAO, or 90-degree LAO with patient in right lateral decubitus (this posi-

tion lowers left diaphragm to provide better visualization of posterior wall).

6. Optionally, a gated acquisition to evaluate wall motion can also be obtained.
   a. Acquire data using conventional 16-frame, multi-gated acquisition mode.
   b. Imaging time increased to 8 to 10 minutes per view.

D. SPECT imaging.
   1. Quality control important.
      a. Uniformity correction—30 million count extrinsic flood/week for 64 × 64 matrix.
      b. Center-of-rotation correction.
      c. Detector alignment.
   2. Protocols.
      a. One-day protocol (Table 7-2).
      b. Two-day protocol.
         (1) Use exercise imaging protocol per 1-day study.
   3. Reconstruction.
      a. Different filter parameters are necessary for rest and stress studies to generate tomograms of comparable image texture because raw images have differing count densities. Same parameters can be used for rest and stress for 2-day protocol. Exact parameters vary with each system.

VI. Teboroxime imaging protocol.
   A. SPECT stress.
      1. Triple-headed camera—acquisition beginning within 2 minutes of injection and continuing for 10 to 16 minutes.
   B. Rest study performed 2 hours later.

VII. Computer-assisted diagnosis (CAID) of cardiac perfusion studies.
   A. Goals of CAID.
      1. Reduce interobserver variability.

Table 7-2 ^{99m}Tc Sestamibi SPECT Imaging Protocol

	Rest	Exercise
Energy window	20% symmetric	Same
Collimator	High-resolution	Same
Orbit	180 degrees	Same
Number/projections	64	Same
Matrix	64 × 64	Same
Time/projection	25 seconds	20 seconds
Total time	30 minutes	25 minutes
Frames/cycle (if gating)	1	8

2. Provide interpretation equal to that of a human observer.
3. Ultimately, increase sensitivity over visual reading.
B. Parameters evaluated by CAID.
1. Identify perfusion defects.
2. Determine whether defects are artifact or real.
3. Differentiate ischemia from infarct.
4. Assign defect to a vascular distribution.
C. Primary techniques to determine whether a segment is abnormal.
1. Compare activity to a normal file (most commonly used).
2. Compare activity in one segment to another.
D. Overview of technique for quantitation of ^{201}Tl and sestamibi scans.
1. Acquire images using special protocol.
2. Process images using CAID program
3. Create circumferential profile of slices.
4. Create temporal washout profile.
5. Compare profiles with normal file.
6. Display results.
E. Image acquisition—extremely important for quantitation that exactly the same protocol be used for each patient.
1. Identical doses.
2. Same camera and computer setup.
3. Same imaging times.
4. Exact repositioning of patient between stress and redistribution.
F. Circumferential profiles.
1. Most programs create a circumferential profile. This is a "map" of the counts at various intervals around the circumference of the cardiac image.
2. Plot 60 radii at 6-degree intervals.
3. Find the pixel with the highest counts in each 6-degree wedge of myocardium.
   a. Problems with using maximal counts.
      (1) Assessment of a segment is based on only one pixel.
      (2) The pixels compared at stress and redistribution may not be the same.
      (3) Defects will be missed if they involve only part of a segment.
      (4) Quality control, since quality control is based on counts in a single pixel.
   b. Mean versus maximal counts.
      (1) Maximal activity 20% to 25% greater than mean.
      (2) Sensitivity for CAD the same.

(3) Specificity improved (94% versus 83%) using mean counts.
G. Normal files.
  1. Based on patients with pretest low likelihood of CAD (1% to 3%).
  2. Anatomic location of segment with maximal counts varies; data are pooled to obtain mean and standard deviation.
  3. Since normal profiles vary between men and women, gender-based normal files should be used.
    a. Women have decreased anterior activity because of breast attenuation.
    b. Men have decreased inferior activity because of diaphragm attenuation.
H. Normalization.
  1. Delayed plot normalized to stress. Maximal-count pixel on stress image is compared to maximum counts on redistribution images. The delayed images are multiplied by the ratio of activity to make them comparable to stress images.
 I. Criteria for abnormality.
  1. Standard deviation of 2.5 below mean, or counts below a range.
  2. Clustering—several contiguous pixels must be abnormal to classify as abnormal; improves statistics.
  3. Size (percentage) of a vascular territory that is flagged as abnormal.
 J. Abnormals—counts fall below the lower limit of normal.
K. Washout profiles (not frequently done with SPECT; more common with planar imaging).
  1. Percentage of thallium that clears over 2 to 4 hours.
  2. Clearance is slower in ischemic tissue.
  3. Why is clearance slower in ischemic tissue?
    a. Initial thallium uptake depends on blood flow.
    b. Washout is due to difference between myocardial and blood concentrations.
  4. Normal washout files:
    a. Women—65%.
    b. Males—57%.
  5. Technical factors that adversely affect the washout profile.
    a. Delayed stress and redistribution scans (imaging times must be precise).
    b. Low count rates.
    c. Reangulation errors between stress and redistribution.
    d. Submaximal exercise.
    e. Arm vein uptake. Patients sometimes show uptake of ^{201}Tl in the vein. The activity can then slowly leak into the blood,

affecting the measured washout rate.
6. Washout results (planar).
   a. Visual analysis—61%.
   b. Quantitative analysis—93%.
7. Washout results—SPECT: No improvement in sensitivity by adding washout analysis to circumferential profile analysis.
L. Polar or bull's-eye plot.
1. Maps 3-D SPECT data to 2-D display.
2. Is the usual way the studies are displayed.
M. Reversibility plot—differentiates infarct from ischemia.
N. Results.
1. Sensitivity—73% to 95%.
2. Specificity—44% to 74%.
   a. Specificity may be lower because of post-test referral bias.
      (1) Positive test goes to cath.
      (2) Negative test does not.
      (3) Results in lower measured specificity.
   b. Normalcy rate is sometimes used in these circumstances.
      (1) Specificity—true-negatives/true-negatives + false-positives.
      (2) Normalcy rate—how frequently test excludes disease in <5% probability of CAD population.
O. Sources of error.
1. Normal variants.
   a. Apical thinning and partial volume averaging can cause a false-positive result.
   b. Displaced apex—if apex is displaced medially or laterally, program may erroneously flag as abnormal.
   c. Hot spots—result from papillary muscles and other unknown causes.
      (1) Since display is normalized to the hottest pixel, a hot spot can cause the remainder of the scan to be "normalized" down to a level that is perceived as abnormal by the program.
2. Gender differences.
   a. Large breast size (more attenuation).
   b. Following mastectomy (less attenuation, changes ratio of anterior/inferior wall).
   c. Male gynecomastia (more atttenuation than expected).
3. Nonischemic cardiac disease.
   a. Left bundle branch block.
   b. Left ventricular hypertrophy.
   c. Dextrorotation or levorotation.
4. Imaging artifacts.
   a. Repositioning errors.

    b. Patient motion.

      (1) Occurs in 10% of patients.

      (2) Movement of only 0.5 to 1 pixel (3 to 6 mm) can produce an artifact.

      (3) Pixel movement of 1+ produces false-positive result in 40% of patients.

    c. Heart creep. Increased excursion of the diaphragm immediately after exercise can cause the inferior wall to move in and out of the tomographic slices making a "defect." It will appear to redistribute, since the patient is breathing normally on delayed images. Can be prevented by waiting approximately 15 minutes after exercise before initiating imaging.

  5. Reconstruction artifacts.

    a. Skewing of axis of reconstruction.

    b. Incorrect apical slice selection—leads to partial-volume averaging.

  6. Camera and computer artifacts.

    a. Center-of-rotation errors.

    b. Nonuniformity.

 P. Thallium stress database not applicable to:

  1. Rest.

  2. Dipyridamole.

  3. ^{99m}Tc agents.

Normal Findings

 I. Rest study—planar.

  A. Right ventricle normally not seen (although 10% to 15% of patients may show faint activity).

  B. See stress study.

 II. Stress study-planar.

  A. Right ventricular activity normally seen on both initial and redistribution images.

  B. Mild inhomogeneity in left ventricle is not uncommon. Variation in counts of 15% to 20% as one goes around circumference of left ventricle is not unusual.

  C. Anterior view.

    1. Reverse C shape (Fig. 7-1).

    2. Frequently, inferior walls show less activity than anterolateral.

    3. Slit-like defect representing normal apical thinning also not uncommon. With these as with all normal variants, the lack of change between stress and redistribution is helpful in differentiating from ischemia (although not helpful in differentiating from infarct).

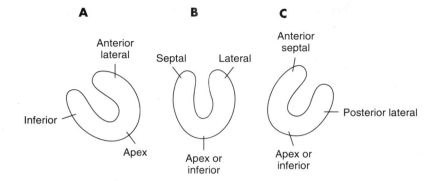

Fig. 7-1 Walls as seen on planar ^{201}Tl scan on, **A**, anterior, **B**, 45-degree left anterior oblique, and **C**, lateral views.

4. Location of defect is helpful in determining vessel involved (Fig. 7-2).
5. In women, breast attenuation may cause artifacts involving anterior wall. Sweeping line across heart divides image into "low count" portion above, and "high count" portion below. By taping breast up out of position, defect will resolve.

D. LAO.

1. In 65% of patients, complete "doughnut" of activity present. In 20%, defect is present due to valve plane oriented 12 o'clock position. In remaining 15%, defect is off 12 o'clock position, usually more laterally.
2. Superior septum frequently shows decreased activity.
3. Apical defect again may be seen.
4. In females, breast may cause decreased activity in upper septum and upper lateral walls.
5. Vascular distribution or all three coronary arteries best laid out in this view.

E. Left lateral.

1. C-shaped area of activity with defect at approximately 2 o'clock position. Defect may rotate down to 3 o'clock position as a normal variant.
2. If patient not imaged in right lateral decubitus position, pseudodefect may occur along posterior wall.

III. SPECT studies.

A. Short-axis views.

1. "Doughnut" of activity seen. Often, decreased activity inferiorly resulting from attentuation of low energy photons.

    a. Artifacts/normal variants.

      (1) As slices approach base of heart, membranous septum

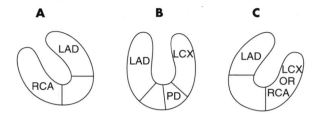

Fig. 7-2 Vascular distribution seen on three views of planar thallium scan. **A,** Anterior; **B,** 40-degree left anterior oblique, and **C,** 60-degree left anterior oblique views. *LAD,* Left anterior descending; *LCX,* left circumflex; *PD,* posterior descending; *RCA,* right coronary artery.

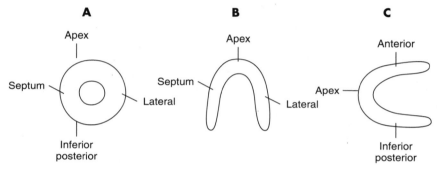

Fig. 7-3 Walls seen on SPECT imaging. **A,** Short axis, **B,** horizontal long axis, and **C,** vertical long axis.

causes asymmetry of activity between septum (decreased activity) and lateral wall. Can be misinterpreted as infarct.
  (2) Gender differences.
    (a) Females may show decreased anterior wall activity because of breast attenuation.
    (b) Males frequently have decreased inferoposterior activity because of diaphragmatic attenuation.
  2. Walls as shown in Fig. 7-3.
B. Vertical long-axis.
  1. Reverse C-shaped activity. May see decreased activity inferoposteriorly.
  2. Walls as shown in Fig. 7-3.
C. Horizontal long-axis.
    a. Artifacts/normal variants.
      (1) Apical thinning.
        (a) Apex can normally be very thin, mimicking a defect.

(2) Displaced apex.
    (a) Apex may be displaced laterally or medially. Do not confuse with defect.
(3) Upper third of septum frequently "absent." This, again, is membranous septum.
(4) May see decreased activity as approach base.

Abnormal Findings

  I. Right ventricular activity at rest.
 II. Cold defect involving left ventricle, which may or may not redistribute.
III. Defect or absence of activity of right ventricle with exercise (right coronary disease).

Diseases

I. Ischemic cardiac disease.
  A. Most common reason for ordering exercise thallium scan.
    1. Sensitivity and specificity for coronary artery disease:
      a. Planar imaging, 75% sensitivity if criteria reversible defects. From 80% to 85% if criteria reversible and nonreversible defects.
      b. Specificity, 95% if reversible defects; 85% to 90% if both reversible and nonreversible defects.
      c. Planar + computer analysis—sensitivity, 90%; specificity falls—degree depends on patient population studied.
      d. SPECT—90+ % sensitivity. Specificity somewhat lower than planar but higher than computer analysis.
    2. Sensitivity for *detection* of coronary artery disease increases from single to multivessel disease.
      a. 73%—1 vessel.
      b. 87%—2 vessels.
      c. 97%—3 vessels.
    3. However, radionuclides tend to *underestimate* extent of coronary disease. When patient develops symptoms of most critical stenosis, exercise stopped. Therefore often see defect only in the more severely affected area. Dipyridamole may be better way to evaluate for multivessel disease.
    4. Sensitivity for determining individual vessels involved (63% overall).
      a. Left anterior descending (74%) and right coronary artery (69%)-best.
      b. Circumflex (38%)-worst. In fact, sensitivities for circumflex so much lower than other vessels, cannot be used to exclude disease in this distribution.

    c. If defects seen in septum and posterolateral walls, *some* evidence for left main disease; however, may be related to distal disease in both vessels.

    d. If fixed defects present, sensitivity for disease in a vascular distribution increases to 100% LAD, 80% right coronary, and 65% circumflex. Note that when prior infarct is in right or circumflex distribution, disease in LAD detected with high sensitivity. But when infarction in LAD distribution, detection of concomitant disease in right or circumflex artery is poor.

5. Specificity varies with patient population. If study performed on patients with low likelihood of CAD, specificity falls significantly.

B. Specific patients that thallium scan is best suited for:

1. Bayesian analysis indicates scan best for patients with approximately 50% pretest probability of having CAD.

    a. If patient has extremely high probability for disease, positive scan confirms what was already clinically thought. Negative scan likely false-negative.

    b. In patients with very low likelihood, negative scan confirms clinical suspicion, positive scan likely false-positive.

2. Positive exercise ECG in absence of chest pain.

    a. These patients have approximately 30% prevalence of CAD.

    b. Presence or lack of ^{201}Tl defects excellent for determining presence or absence of coronary disease.

3. Positive ECG in patients with nonanginal chest pain.

    a. Only slightly higher likelihood of having CAD than group of patients who are asymptomatic.

4. Patient in whom chest pain occurs during exercise without ECG changes.

5. Patients with abnormal baseline ECG that presents problems interpreting stress tracing.

    a. Arrhythmia.

    b. Left bundle-branch block.

    c. Left ventricular hypertrophy.

6. Patients taking medications that alter ECG tracing.

    a. Digitalis.

7. Patients in whom fatigue causes submaximal exercise study rates.

    a. Summary of four studies indicates sensitivity of thallium of 91%, specificity of 86% in this group. Therefore, appears thallium more sensitive than treadmill-ECG studies in face of inadequate exercise. Note discussion in "Technique" section, however.

8. Atypical chest pain.
   a. Approximately 50% likelihood of CAD.
   b. Sensitivity and specificity of treadmill ECG lower than stress thallium in these patients.
9. Evaluation of extent of CAD.
   a. Left main disease and multivessel disease have poor prognosis. Also, may be considered for bypass grafting.
   b. Sensitivity for detecting CAD with multivessel disease increases. However, extent of disease is frequently underestimated.
   c. Left main disease may be suspected if defects found in distribution of septum and posterolateral wall. However, there is some question about specificity, and sensitivity is only 68%. Multiple defects in all three distributions do correlate very well with triple-vessel disease.
10. Evaluation of functional significance of known anatomic abnormalities.
    a. Angiography gives anatomic size of lesion. Thallium gives physiologic significance.
    b. Lesion with less than 50% to 70% narrowing may be flow limiting if:
       (1) Of sufficient length.
       (2) Eccentric.
       (3) In series with other insignificant stenoses.
    c. One-vessel disease.
       (1) Presence of reversible abnormality in regions supplied by vessel with borderline narrowing is extremely strong evidence that a lesion is hemodynamically significant.
       (2) Absence of stress-induced abnormality, however, only moderately reliable for predicting absence of hemodynamic significance.
       (3) Addition of quantitative analysis appears to improve sensitivity.
    d. Multivessel disease.
       (1) Absence of development of defect in a borderline lesion with a second significant lesion not helpful in excluding hemodynamically significant borderline lesion.
       (2) Dipyridamole may be better than exercise.
       (3) Quantitative analysis again helpful in these cases.
11. Assessment of functional significance of collateral coronary arteries.
    a. Functional significance of collateral vessels not evaluated well by angiographic technique.

      b. Lack of development of thallium defect good evidence of efficacy of collaterals.

      c. Development of a defect indicates that collaterals are inadequate for preventing regional hypoperfusion.

  12. Assessment of myocardial viability.

      a. Difficult with coronary angiography to assess myocardial viability.

      b. Wall motion abnormalities may occur even in viable tissue.

      c. Interventional ventriculography effective to assess viability, but invasive.

      d. Uptake of thallium in region excellent evidence of viability.

      e. Many perform exercise with redistribution to evaluate viability. If rest only performed, "redistribution" images must be performed. Has been shown that high-grade narrowing of coronary artery in absence of infarction may cause resting regional myocardial hypoperfusion.

      f. Studies indicate routine (^{201}Tl) scans with 4-hour redistribution imaging underestimates cardiac viability by 30% to 50%.

        (1) Reinjection of 1 mCi just before routine redistribution images significantly improves detection of reversibility.

        (2) Technique logistically superior to 24-hour imaging.

        (3) Some studies indicate that for maximal sensitivity for viable tissue, a routine redistribution scan or 24-hour imaging must be performed, *in addition to* reinjection imaging.

  13. Evaluation of bypass graft patency.

      a. If abnormal region preoperatively becomes normal postoperatively, indicates patent bypass graft.

      b. If normal region preoperatively becomes abnormal postoperatively, region associated with occluded bypass graft or progression native coronary disease in ungrafted vessel.

      c. If no change in region between pre- and postoperative state, cannot determine whether bypass graft patent.

      d. Dipyridamole appears useful for evaluating patency. May be used in immediate postoperative period.

II. Myocardial infarction.

  A. Acute.

    1. Thallium scan may be used for diagnosis of acute myocardial infarction.

    2. Sensitivity depends on:

      a. Timing.

        (1) First 6 hours after onset of infarction, 100%. High sen-

sitivity is result of periinfarction ischemia contributing to size of defect.

    (2) After 24 hours, sensitivity 75%.

  b. Type.

    (1) Transmural—85% to 100% sensitivity.

    (2) Nontransmural—50%.

    (3) Anterior—100% sensitivity.

    (4) Inferior—85%.

  3. Specificity.

    a. May see rest defects in patients with unstable angina. Delayed imaging may show reperfusion.

    b. In patient without unstable angina, still cannot differentiate between recent infarction and past event.

  B. Old infarction.

    1. Sensitivity for old infarction approximately 70%. Reasons for lower sensitivity are:

    a. Small size of infarction.

    b. Scar retraction with time.

    c. Overlying normal areas obscuring infarction.

III. ^{99m}Tc sestamibi.

  A. Interpretation similar to ^{201}Tl.

  B. Clinical comparison of ^{99m}Tc sestamibi and ^{201}Tl.

    1. Numerous clinical studies comparing ^{201}Tl and ^{99m}Tc have been performed.

    2. In U.S. multicenter trial of 278 patients:

    a. Total agreement on 92% of perfusion defects and 83% of uptake patterns (normal, reversible, nonreversible).

    b. Sestamibi not statistically different: ^{99m}Tc—89%; ^{201}Tl—90%.

    c. Specificities also similar.

    d. Normalcy rate (true negative rate in individuals with less than 5% likelihood of coronary artery disease)—81%.

IV. ^{99m}Tc teboroxime.

  A. Phase III trial of 177 patients, including both planar and SPECT images for diagnosis of coronary artery disease.

  B. Sensitivity 83%; specificity 81%.

^{99M}Tc PYROPHOSPHATE IMAGING

Anatomy

I. Myocardial infarction.

  A. Almost all infarcts involve LV.

    1. Anterior wall and septum most often involved, since LAD most commonly affected vessel.

2. Inferior wall and posterior third of septum is second most common site.
3. Right ventricle involved in 25% to 50% of patients with inferior wall infarction—rare to be involved without LV infarction.
B. Coronary thrombosis present in half of infarcts. Intramural hemorrhage in 40%. Most frequently occluded arteries are:
   1. LAD (56%).
   2. Right coronary (25%).
   3. Circumflex (14%).
C. Coronary thrombosis usually associated with transmural infarction, although thrombi might be result rather than the cause of infarction. Coronary artery spasm may be primary cause of infarction in at least some of these patients.
D. Coronary thrombi probably *not* cause of infarction in patients with sudden death *or* subendocardial infarction.
E. Infarction may be classified by degree of thickness of necrosis.
   1. Transmural, or Q-wave—full-thickness myocardial wall.
   2. Nontransmural, or non–Q-wave—less than full thickness of wall.
   3. Subendocardial infarction—less than one-half thickness of wall.

Physiology

I. Myocardial infarction.
   A. Microscopic changes in myocardial cells seen as early as 5 to 10 minutes after ligation of coronary arteries in animals.
   B. In large transmural infarctions, there is reduced blood flow to center of infarction, particularly in endocardium. Blood flow to periphery of infarction is reduced much less.
II. Technetium 99m pyrophosphate—determinants of uptake in infarction.
   A. Blood flow.
      1. ^{99m}Tc pyrophosphate must reach damaged tissue to be taken up.
         a. Highest concentration of ^{99m}Tc pyrophosphate occurs when local blood flow reduced by 20% to 40%.
         b. As flow further reduced, concentration falls in regions of severely reduced flow.
         c. Concentration of pyrophosphate greater in epicardial than endocardial segments at same blood flow rate.
         d. Pyrophosphate ratio of 18 to 20 infarcted tissue/normal myocardium possible.
   B. Extraction.
      1. Extraction fraction does *not* increase with decreased flow; thus, total amount tracer extracted decreases at low flow.

C. Calcium influx.
  1. Key role in ^{99m}Tc pyrophosphate binding in acute infarction.
  2. Intracellular calcium deposition occurs in infarcted tissue.
  3. Calcium forms calcium phosphate and is present in three forms in cell:
      a. Amorphous—distributed uniformly through cell.
      b. Crystalline.
      c. Hydroxyapatite—primarily in mitochondria.
  4. Pyrophosphate binds to both amorphous and hydroxyapatite deposits.
  5. Although not linear, ^{99m}Tc pyrophosphate concentration parallels calcium phosphate concentration.
D. Necrotic tissue.
  1. Pyrophosphate labels acutely *necrotic* myocardium.
  2. Even in diseases other than acute myocardial infarction, such as unstable angina, histopathologic examination has indicated multifocal lesions of necrosis and myocytolysis. Similar explanations for uptake in ventricular aneurysm.
III. Timing.
  A. Earliest uptake 4 hours after coronary artery occlusion.
  B. Peak uptake at 48 hours.
  C. Gradually diminish over next 5 to 7 days.
  D. Time course varies depending on:
    1. Size of infarction—due to markedly diminished perfusion in center of infarction. The larger the infarct, the longer the time for peak uptake. In addition, will fade more slowly because of continuing tissue necrosis.
    2. Extension of infarction—which causes increase and prolongation of uptake.

Technique

  I. Prepare ^{99m}Tc pyrophosphate such that reduced hydrolized technetium less than 5%, free technetium less than 1%.
 II. Inject 20 mCi of pyrophosphate intravenously.
III. Wait 2 to 4 hours and begin imaging.
IV. Using high-resolution collimator and standard field camera, obtain 400,000 counts per view. Views obtained:
  A. Anterior.
  B. 35-degree LAO.
  C. 70-degree LAO.
  D. Left lateral.
 V. SPECT
  A. 128 × 128 image matrix with a hardware zoom of 1.3 to 1.5.

B. 360-degree rotation.

C. 64 to 128 stops for a total acquisition time of 30 minutes.

D. Reconstruction and filtering are system dependent.

Normal Scan

I. Since ^{99m}Tc pyrophosphate is a bone agent, sternum and rib activity present.

II. If no blood pool activity present, no evidence of soft tissue seen in region of myocardium.

III. If blood pool present, faint activity (see below) may be seen diffusely in cardiac region. Delayed imaging can be helpful.

IV. Linear activity may be present in costal cartilages, simulating inferior wall infarction.

V. Kidney activity present, may be misinterpreted as myocardial activity. Location, low in chest/abdomen, should differentiate.

Abnormal Scans

I. Increased uptake in region of myocardium.

II. Grading system as follows:

A. 0 = no activity.

B. 1+ = minimal activity because of blood pool or chest wall activity.

C. 2+ = definite myocardial activity but less than bone.

D. 3+ = activity equal to bone.

E. 4+ = activity greater than bone.

III. Activity 0 to 1+ indicates negative scan. Activity 2+ or greater indicates positive scan.

IV. Eighty percent of patients with acute transmural infarction have 3+ or 4 +; 20% have 2+.

V. Location of activity on oblique views useful in localizing wall involved.

VI. Diffuse uptake may be sign of subendocardial infarction. Difficult to differentiate from blood pool.

Diseases

I. Acute myocardial infarction.

A. Sensitivity depends on timing. If imaged between 48 and 72 hours after infarction:

1. Transmural infarction—95%.

2. Nontransmural infarction—80%.

3. Sensitivity highest for anterior infarctions, lowest for inferior wall infarction (because not seen en face).

4. SPECT improves sensitivity.

B. Specificity.

     1. Approximately 80+%.
     2. Specificity improves as activity increases from 2+ to 4+.
     3. Specificity significantly greater for focal accumulation than for diffuse uptake.
     4. Previous myocardial infarction–persistently postive scan—occurs in 20% of MIs.
  C. Pyrophosphate scan especially useful in:
    a. Patients in whom enzymes or ECG do not allow diagnosis.
      a. Those with ECG abnormalities.
      b. Infarcts more than 48 hours old, for which CK-MB fractions can be unreliable.
      c. Patients who recently have undergone cardiac surgery/cardioversion.

II. Perioperative infarction.
  A. New Q waves following bypass graft surgery do not necessarily indicate perioperative infarction.
  B. CK-MB isoenzyme fraction may normally show some elevation following cardiac surgery.
  C. Pyrophosphate both highly sensitive and specific for diagnosis of perioperative infarction.
  D. Helpful to obtain baseline pyrophosphate scan on patients undergoing open heart surgery, since they may have persistently positive scan from prior infarctions.

III. Right ventricular infarction.
  A. About 25% to 50% of patients with inferoposterior LV infarction have concomitant RV infarction.
  B. Diagnosis difficult to establish by enzyme or ECG, because both are abnormal due to LV infarction.
  C. May show characteristic "W" lesion on LAO, due to inferior wall, lower septum, and RV uptake.

IV. Prognosis.
  A. Pyrophosphate can be used to size infarction.
    1. Studies indicate larger size infarctions are associated with poor prognosis.
    2. Pattern of uptake also helpful for prognosis. A "doughnut" pattern indicates significantly increased mortality.
      a. Pattern due to extensive myocardial necrosis with poor blood flow preventing pyrophosphate from entering center of infarction.
      b. Almost always in LAD distribution.
      c. Associated with large infarction; hence, poor prognosis.

V. Amyloidosis.
  A. *Bi*ventricular uptake specific sign of cardiac amyloidosis.

VI. Uptake has been described in other diseases, including:
   A. Adriamycin cardiotoxicity.
   B. Radiation cardiotoxicity.
   C. Pericarditis.
   D. Myocarditis.
   E. Myocardial contusion.
   F. Cardiac injury resulting from repeated cardioversion.

GATED BLOOD POOL IMAGING (MUGA)
Radiopharmaceuticals

I. ^{99m}Tc human serum albumin (^{99m}Tc HSA).
   A. Original material used for blood pool studies. Now largely replaced by ^{99m}Tc-labeled red blood cells (RBCs).
   B. Problem with HSA—leaks from vascular space, results in lower target-to-background ratios than ^{99m}Tc-labeled RBCs.
II. ^{99m}Tc-labeled RBCs.
   A. Most commonly labeled for gated blood pool studies.
   B. Several labeling techniques.
      1. In vitro technique.
         a. Commonly used technique.
         b. Exact technique varies with commercial kit.
            (1) Example: Draw 1 to 3 ml of blood into tube containing heparin or ACD.
            (2) Add to reaction vial containing stannous chloride. Portion of stannous ion in vial crosses red cell membrane and accumulates intracellularly. Allow reaction for 5 minutes.
            (3) Add sodium hypochlorite. This oxidizes extracellular stannous ion. Note: Hypochlorite does not cross red cell membrane.
            (4) Add citric acid, sodium citrate, and dextrose solution to sequester any residual extracellular stannous ion, rendering it more available for oxidation by sodium hypochlorite.
            (5) Add 10 to 100 mCi of pertechnetate, and incubate for 20 minutes.
            (6) Inject within 30 minutes of preparation.
      2. In vivo.
         a. Cold stannous pyrophosphate injected IV.
         b. Fifteen minutes later, 15 to 30 mCi ^{99m}Tc pertechnetate injected.
         c. Labeling process occurs within intravascular space. ^{99m}Tc binds rapidly to globin portion of hemoglobin molecule.

     d. Labeling efficiency 80% to 90%.

     e. Important to mix vial of cold stannous pyrophosphate just before injection to minimize potential for chemical oxidation of stannous ion via introduction of air into vial.

  3. Modified in vivo.

     a. Less common technique.

     b. Has improved labeling efficiency compared with in vivo technique. Labeling efficiencies of 98% possible. This reduces free pertechnetate in GI tract and interstitium of lung.

     c. Labeling performed in closed system attached to patient's vein.

     d. Butterfly needle placed in vein with extension tube and three-way stop cock at end.

     e. Cold stannous pyrophosphate administered IV.

     f. Fifteen minutes later, line flushed with heparanized saline, 5 to 10 ml of blood withdrawn into syringe containing 15 to 30 mCi of ^{99m}Tc pertechnetate with small amount anticoagulant.

     g. Syringe gently agitated for 10 minutes.

     h. Labeled RBCs reinjected via butterfly.

C. Dose

  1. Standard adult dose.

     a. Twenty to 30 mCi of pertechnetate. Best to use higher dose with exercise studies, since those acquired for only 2 to 3 minutes per exercise stage.

  2. Minimum pediatric dose.

     a. Two to 3 mCi. Dose can be calculated using 200 µCi/kg.

D. Repeated imaging can be performed following labeling for up to 12 hours.

Technique

I. Multigated studies.

  A. Uses ECG as physiologic synchronizer or "gate." Detects and uses R wave as reference point of electrical (which reflects mechanical) end diastole. Cardiac cycle then divided into frames.

  B. Originally, two data frames collected: One at R wave for end diastole and one at end of T wave for end systole.

  C. In current approach, data collection initiated at R wave, and 12 to 64 consecutive frames recorded throughout cardiac cycle.

  D. Data acquisition.

    1. Frame model.

      a. Most common data acquisition technique.

b. Data from each cardiac cycle added to counts from previous cycles already stored in each frame. Once adequate data density obtained, an "average" beat is obtained.

c. Problem with technique: ectopic beats, such as premature ventricular contractions (PVCs), which vary in beat length and ejection fraction, are averaged in with "normal" beats.

d. To prevent this, beat reject software can be used. The RR interval is calculated for normal sinus rhythm. Any beats with significant variation (20% variation in beat length) are rejected. This is done by saving data in buffer in computer and checking it *before* adding it to data already collected.

2. List mode.

a. Less commonly performed technique. Requires much greater storage capacity on computer and much more processing time.

b. The x and y coordinates of each scintillation event are stored separately in computer memory in serial manner. Time markers and R-wave markers also placed, i.e., location, clock time, and time relative to R-wave of each count recorded.

c. Once all data collected, operator can determine which beats are used in the study. Especially useful for patients with severe arrhythmias (Fig. 7-4).

E. Temporal framing rate important. If too few frames used to acquire data, will average peaks and valleys of emptying curve; thus, calculated ejection fraction will be spuriously low. Typically, framing rates used are:

1. Rest—35 to 50 msec/frame.
2. Exercise—20 to 30 msec/frame.
3. To determine filling rates, etc., from emptying curves, higher temporal resolution required. Usually 10- to 20-msec intervals.

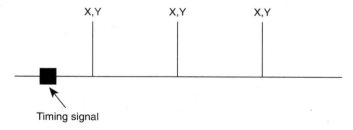

Fig. 7-4   List mode acquisition with timing marker and location of each event.

F. Data typically acquired with matrix size of 64 × 64 pixels.

G. Outline of multigated acquisition.

    1. Rest.

        a. Patient given nothing by mouth for 4 to 8 hours before examination.

        b. Red cells labeled as outlined in radiopharmaceutical section.

        c. Place ECG leads. Make sure strong R-wave obtained.

        d. Set computer for 16-frame acquisition, 64 × 64 matrix.

        e. Obtain ECG and determine average beat length. Set beat reject software for ±20%.

        f. Using standard-field-of-view camera equipped with general all-purpose collimator, perform anterior, 45-degree LAO, left lateral, 30-degree LPO views.

        g. A 20% window set is used and centered over 140 keV.

        h. Data should be acquired for minimum of 200 counts per pixel over LV (approximately 200,000 to 350,000 counts/frame).

        i. On LAO view, can use 10-degree caudal tilt to better separate LV from left atrium. As alternative, can use 30-degree slant-hole collimator.

    2. Exercise.

        a. Patient placed on bicycle (usually recumbent).

        b. Baseline LAO view obtained.

        c. Patient taken through graded exercise on bicycle with 3-minute acquisitions at each exercise level.

        d. Postexercise (recovery) images obtained following completion of exercise.

II. First-pass studies.

A. Radiopharmaceuticals.

    1. ^{99m}Tc pertechnetate.

    2. ^{99m}Tc DTPA or ^{99m}Tc sulfur colloid are preferred if multiple repeat studies are anticipated, such as resting and exercise.

    3. Short-lived agents also used.

        a. ^{195m}Au—30-second half-life.

        b. ^{191m}Ir—4.9-second half-life.

        c. ^{178}Ta—9.3-minute half-life.

    4. Right ventricular ejection fraction.

        a. Diffusable tracers such as xenon or krypton 81m can be used.

    5. Small volume with high specific activity recommended. Typically, 10- to 25-mCi technetium agent used in less than 1 ml.

    6. Injected rapidly followed by 20-ml saline flush through basilic vein in antecubital fossa. Even better to use central catheter.

    7. Since count rates obtained with this technique can be extremely high, multicrystal gamma camera is theoretically

best. Can handle counting rates of 450,000 counts per second without significant deadtime losses. Conventional single crystal camera, on other hand, can only handle 60 to 100,000 counts per second.
   8. Acquisition can be nongated, gated, or list-mode.
   9. Patient may be positioned anteriorly, although RAO view provides the maximum separation of left atrium from LV and is often preferred.

Data Analysis

I. Visual analysis.
   A. To improve appearance, gated studies are frequently filtered.
      1. Spatial smoothing—each surrounding pixel around an individual pixel is examined and counts are averaged using a weighting algorithm.
      2. Temporal smoothing—counts in pixel frame before and after are averaged.
   B. Ejection fraction.
      1. Background area drawn along posterolateral wall of ventricle. Approximately 2 pixels from the wall, several pixels wide, 5 to 6 pixels long.
      2. Background then subtracted from image.
      3. Edge detection.
         a. Manual.
            (1) Ventricle is outlined at end diastole. End systolic frame then determined and outlined manually.
            (2) Ejection fraction =

$$\frac{\text{end diastolic counts} - \text{end sytolic counts}}{\text{end diastolic counts}}$$

            after correction for background.

         b. Computer—using variety of algorithms, determines edges and automatically generates ejection fraction.

Normal Study

I. Visual analysis.
   A. Activity representing RBCs in spleen and liver seen inferiorly on all views.
   B. Black line separating heart from lung and hepatic activity normally present because of fat. If extremely thick, pericardial effusion should be considered.
   C. Aorta, pulmonary outflow tract, left and right pulmonary arteries visible. Normally smooth without dilatation.

D. Right atrium—best seen on anterior view. Depending on rotation of heart, may be more prominent in some normals. If there is a question of right atrial enlargement, check RV size and function, since isolated right atrial enlargement is rare.

E. Left atrium-seen on LAO and left lateral views. Normally smaller than LV. Large variation in shape. In atrial fibrillation, may not appear to contract.

F. Right ventricle-on LAO view, great overlap between right atrium and ventricle. Because of pattern of contraction of RV, may appear to be hypokinetic even in normals on this view. Normally contracts in synchrony with LV. With bundle-branch block, etc., will show delayed contraction.

G. Left ventricle-because of thickness of wall, will see black line representing wall on LAO view. May see defect in superolateral margin on the LAO corresponding to papillary muscles. On left lateral, posteromedial papillary muscle can result in indentation in inferior surface of LV at junction of inferior and apical segments.

II. Ejection fraction.

A. LV EF—50% to 65% normal. RV EF—using gated technique, usually higher than left side. This is due to technique, *not* physiology.

Diseases

I. Ischemic coronary artery disease.

A. Findings.

1. Rest.

a. Wall motion abnormalities—indicate past myocardial infarction as sign of coronary disease. Ischemia almost never results in wall motion abnormality at rest, similar to lack of thallium defects at rest.

b. Ejection fraction—may be decreased if past myocardial infarction; otherwise, normal.

2. Exercise.

a. Wall motion abnormalities-development of wall motion abnormalities most specific sign of CAD. Unfortunately, sensitivity significantly less than fall in EF (see below).

b. Ejection fraction.

(1) Normal—5 EF unit increase with exercise.

(2) Abnormal—fall in EF best sign. Increase less than 5 units or no change also abnormal, but not as strong evidence of CAD.

2. Sensitivity—varies in literature—approximately 85% to 90%.

a. Highest for triple-vessel disease.

        b. Magnitude of fall in EF increases as severity of coronary artery disease worsens. *However,* in individual patient, LV dysfunction represents *severity* of transient ischemia rather than *number* of diseased coronary arteries involved. Single critical LAD lesion may result in same fall in EF as triple-vessel disease with less significant stenoses.

    3. Specificity is lower.

        a. A number of processes result in abnormal responses to exercise other than CAD. In normal persons these include:

            (1) Age > 60 years—may see flat or even fall without CAD. Apparently related to decreased exercise reserve with age.

            (2) Females—may not augment EF.

            (3) Those with elevated resting LV EF such as from increased sympathetic tone associated with anxiety—frequently show flat response. Many consider this "normal."

            (4) Supine exercise—shows less increase in EF than upright exercise.

        d. Decreased exercise reserve occurs in diseases other than CAD.

            (1) Valvular heart disease.

            (2) Left bundle-branch block.

            (3) Myocarditis.

            (4) Non-ischemic cardiomyopathy.

            (5) Mitral valve prolapse.

            (6) Hypertension—controversial.

II. Myocardial infarction (MI).

  A. Findings.

    1. Regional wall motion abnormalities. Note: Patients with inferior wall infarcts may show posterobasilar segmental defect seen only on left lateral or LPO.

    2. Varying degrees of ventricular dilatation.

    3. Reduced LV EF (may be normal, however).

  B. Anterior MI exhibits greater depression in LV EF than does inferior infarction.

  C. Right ventricular infarction occurs almost exclusively in patients with inferior wall MI. 25% to 50% patients with inferior wall MI show right ventricular dysfunction.

  D. Left ventricular aneurysms.

    1. True aneurysm—consists of all normal coverings.

      a. Findings.

(1) Localized bulge in left ventricular contour.
(2) Paradoxical wall motion.
(3) Wide mouth.
(4) Usually located anteriorly or anteroapically.
2. False aneurysm—rupture of heart with bleeding. Bound only by epicardium.
a. Findings.
(1) Abnormal bulge in left ventricular contour.
(2) Paradoxical wall motion.
(3) *Narrow* neck.
(4) Usually located *posterolaterally.*
3. Sensitivity for aneurysms-90% to 95%.
E. Rest and exercise studies helpful in determining prognosis after MI. Significantly lowered EF (<35%) at rest indicative of high 6-month mortality rate.
III. Valvular heart disease.
A. Quantitation of valvular regurgitation
1. Normally, the left and right ventricular stroke volumes are equal. In patients with aortic or mitral insufficiency, left-sided stroke volume greater than right. This can be used to quantitate regurgitation.
2. Technique.
a. Rest MUGA performed in LAO projection.
b. End-systolic image subtracted from end-diastolic image. This yields stroke volume image.
c. Number of counts in left and right ventricles obtained.
d. Stroke volume index = left ventricular counts/right ventricular counts.
3. The greater the ratio, the greater the degree of regurgitation.
4. Note that in normal persons, index may be slightly greater than 1 due to technical problems with technique.
B. Determining optimal time for valve replacement.
1. In left-sided valvular regurgitation, dilatation and hypertrophy develops. This reflected by increased left ventricular EDV and ESV. After years of volume overload, left ventricular contractility decreases, resulting in left ventricular failure.
2. Unfortunately, LVEF at rest is not a sensitive indicator of the state of left ventricular function with valvular regurgitation because of changes in LV preload and afterload that affect LV EF determination. This results in patients with normal preoperative resting LV EF to show reduced EF (with elevated LV ESV) postoperatively.

3. A more sensitive indicator of diminished LV contractile reserve in patients with diseases such as aortic insufficiency is LV EF response to exercise. Perform serial determinations. When patient develops abnormal response to exercise, indicates development of significant ventricular dysfunction but before more chronic and severe changes occur.

IV. Doxorubicin (Adriamycin) cardiotoxicity.
   A. Can result in congestive heart failure.
   B. Usually no significant toxicity below cumulative dose of 350 mg/sq m. With high doses, greater than 550 mg/sq m, approximately one third develop cardiotoxicity, although response is partially idiosyncratic.
   C. Can use MUGA to evaluate for early signs of cardiotoxicity so that therapy can be stopped before development of failure.
   D. Perform first MUGA at cumulative dose 300 mg/sq m.
   E. Beginning at 350 to 450 mg/sq m, repeat examination before each dose.
   F. Abnormalities defined as:
      1. Mild cardiotoxicity.
         a. Absolute decrease in LV $\geq$ 10 EF units.
         b. Absolute EF >45%.
      2. Moderate cardiotoxicity.
         a. Absolute decrease LV EF $\geq$15%.
         b. Absolute LV EF $\leq$45%.
      3. Severe cardiotoxicity.
         a. LV EF $\leq$30%.
   G. Mild cardiotoxicity is early warning of subsequent problems, but therapy can be continued.
   H. Moderate cardiotoxicity indicates doxorubicin therapy should be discontinued. Follow-up studies obtained 1 and 3 months later. Depending on these results, may be possible to cautiously reinstitute therapy.

V. Cardiomyopathy.
   A. Findings.
      1. Diffuse wall motion abnormalities.
      2. Dilated LV.
      3. Decreased EF.
   B. Normal right ventricular function in face of decreased LV function and more focal wall motion abnormalities is *some* evidence of ischemic cardiomyopathy rather than idiopathic. Bilateral (LV + RV) dysfunction more likely nonischemic cardiomyopathy.
   C. Some studies have shown a more normal response to exercise with nonischemic cardiomyopathy.

VI. Asymmetrical septal hypertrophy.
  A. Findings.
    1. Small ventricle.
    2. Thickened septum.
    3. Hyperdynamic wall motion.
    4. Elevated EF.
VII. Chronic obstructive pulmonary disease (COPD).
  A. Can measure biventricular function to determine if patient's symptoms due to worsening COPD or left ventricular failure.
  B. Findings in COPD.
    1. Right ventricular enlargement.
    2. Displacement of LV superiorly and laterally.
    3. Diffuse hypokinesis of RV.
    4. Diminished RV EF.
    5. LV EF usualy normal unless cardiac disease present.
VIII. Shunt analysis.
  A. Left-to-right shunts can be diagnosed and quantitated using first-pass technique.
  B. Computer analysis of pulmonary time-activity curve is done.
  C. Initial portion of primary peak of pulmonary time-activity curve is used to predict shape of remainder of curve, assuming no recirculation. Curve determined by gamma variant (or fit using simpler techniques) is subtracted from original raw data.
  D. Resulting curve then again fit with gamma variant. Area underneath this second curve represents shunt blood flow. Area under first gamma variant fit is equal to pulmonary blood flow; therefore, using the integrated areas, one can determine QP/QS ratio.
  E. Technique accurate in range of 1.2 to 3.0 pulmonary-to-systemic flow ratios. Ratios < 1.2 cannot be differentiated from normal. Ratios > 3 result in flat pulmonary curve that cannot be analyzed.
  F. Since left ventricular dysfunction can affect pulmonary time-activity curve, EF determination should also be performed.

POSITRON EMISSION TOMOGRAPHY

I. Radiopharmaceuticals.
  A. Rubidium-82.
    1. Myocardial flow marker similar to thallium.
    2. Produced by strontium-82/rubidium-82 generator. On-site cyclotron not necessary.
    3. Physical half-life of 76 seconds allows repeat blood flow measurements within short time intervals.
  B. Nitrogen-13 ammonia.
    1. Myocardial blood flow marker.
    2. Cyclotron-produced.

   3. Tracer avidly extracted by myocardial tissue and retained in form of glutamine.
   4. Physical half-life of 10 minutes.
   5. Excellent image quality with high contrast between heart and surrounding lung and blood pool activity. However, prominent liver uptake can impair evaluation of inferior wall of heart.
 C. Oxygen-15 water.
   1. Myocardial blood flow marker.
   2. Cyclotron-produced.
   3. Physical half-life of 2 minutes.
   4. Diffuses across membranes. However, residual time in cell is short; quickly equilibrates between tissue and vascular space.
 D. Fluorine-18 FDG.
   1. Marker of tissue viability.
   2. Cyclotron-produced.
   3. In fasting state carbohydrates play a minor role in myocardial substrate metabolism.
   4. In presence of ischemia, heart reduces oxidation of long-chain fatty acids and relies on glucose for ATP production.
 II. Technique.
  A. Pharmacologic stress primarily used.
  B. Visual, semiquantitative, and quantitative techniques all used for evaluation.
III. Uses.
  A. Diagnosis of CAD.
   1. Comparisons of PET with SPECT indicate a 10% to 15% diagnostic gain with PET.
   2. Specificity also higher, reflecting improved attenuation correction provided by PET. Soft tissue attenuation in SPECT can be misdiagnosed as an abnormality.
  B. Viability.
   1. PET offers significant improvement over ^{201}Tl in determining tissue viability if routine thallium study performed. If patient reinjected with ^{201}Tl for redistribution, results are more similar.
   2. Technique.
     a. Nitrogen-13 ammonia study performed.
     b. Fluorine-18 FDG study performed.
   3. Interpretation.
     a. Decreased nitrogen-13 ammonia (decreased flow) but increased fluorine-18 FDG (increased glucose metabolism)—viable tissue.
     b. Decreased nitrogen-13 ammonia and decreased fluorine-18 FDG—scar.

SUGGESTED READINGS

Alexander J, Daainiak N, Berger H, et al: Serial assessment of dioxorubicin cardiotoxicity with quantitative radionuclide angiocardiography. *New Engl J Med* 1979; 300:278-283.

Beller GA, Watson DD: Physiological basis of myocardial perfusion imaging with the ^{99m}Tc agents. *Semin Nucl Med* 1991; 21:173-181.

Berger HJ, Gottschalk A, Zaret BL: Radionuclide assessment of left and right ventricular performance. *Radiol Clin North Am* 1980; 18:441-466.

Berger H, Zaret BL: Nuclear cardiology: Medical progress. *New Engl J Med* 1981; 305:799-807, 855-865.

Berger HJ, Zaret BL: Radionuclide assessment of cardiovascular performance. In Freeman L (ed): *Clinical scintillation imaging,* ed. 3. New York, Grune & Stratton, 1984, pp 363-479.

Berger HJ, Zaret BL, Berman DS, et al: Cardiac imaging. In Freeman LM (ed): *Freeman and Johnson's clinical radionuclide imaging.* New York, Grune & Stratton, 1984, p. 363.

Berman DS, Kiat H, VanTrain K, et al: ^{99m}Tc sestamibi in the assessment of chronic coronary artery disease. *Semin Nucl Med* 1991; 21:190-212.

Dehmer GJ, Firth BG, Hillis LD, et al: Nongeometric determination of right ventricular volumes for equilibrium blood pool scans. *Am J Cardiol* 1982; 49:78-84.

DePuey EG, (ed): *Myocardial imaging with ^{99m}Tc sestamibi: A workbook.* DuPont Radiopharmaceuticals, 1991.

Gibbons RJ: ^{99m}Tc sestamibi in the assessment of acute myocardial infarction. *Semin Nucl Med* 1991; 21:213-222.

Johnson LL: Clinical experience with ^{99m}Tc teboroxime. *Semin Nucl Med* 1991; 21:182-189.

Maddox DE, Wynne J, Uren R, et al: Regional ejection fraction: A quantitative radionuclide index of regional left ventricular performance. *Circulation* 1979; 59:1001-1009.

McClees EC, Fajman W, Meizlish JL, et al: Cardiovascular nuclear medicine. In *New concepts of cardiac imaging.* Boston, GK Hall, 1985, pp 97-114.

Meizlish JL, Berger HJ, Plankey JP, et al: Functional left ventricular aneurysm formation following acute anterior transmural myocardial infarction: incidence, natural history and prognostic implications *New Engl J Med* 1984; 311:1001-1006.

Schwaiger M, Hutchins GD: Evaluation of coronary artery disease with positron-emission tomography. *Semin Nucl Med* 1992; 22:210-223.

Van Answegen A, Alderson PO, Nickoloff EL, et al: Temporal resolution requirements for left ventricular time-activity curves. *Radiology* 1980; 135:165-170.

Wackers FJ, Berger HJ, Johnstone DE, et al: Multiple gated cardiac blood pool imaging for left ventricular ejection fraction: Validation of the technique and assessment of variability. *Am J Cardiol* 1979; 43:1159-1166.

Zaret BL, Battler A, Berger HJ, et al: Nuclear cardiology: Report of International Society and Federation of Cardiology and World Health Organization Task Force. *Circulation* 1984; 70:768A-781A.

8

Hematologic Imaging

RADIOLABELED LEUKOCYTES
Physiology

I. Leukocytes—heterogeneous group of nucleated cells that perform different functions. As a group they act to protect host from hazards, such as infection and neoplasia, and assist in repair of damaged tissue.

II. Leukocytes spend only small fraction of life in peripheral blood, using it for transportation to sites where needed.

III. Circulating leukocyte pool composed of:
   A. Neutrophils—59%.
   B. Lymphocytes—34%.
   C. Monocytes—4%.
   D. Eosinophils—3%.
   E. Basophils—0.5%.

IV. Neutrophils.
   A. Life cycle—2 weeks.
   B. Granulocytes in peripheral blood are divided between:
      1. Circulating granulocyte pool—44% of blood leukocytes—cells can be recovered.
      2. Marginated pool—56%—temporarily sequestered in capillaries or adherent to endothelial surface of other vessels.
      3. Dynamic equilibrium exists between two pools. Cells move from marginated to circulating pool with:
         a. Physical exercise.
         b. Epinephrine administration.
         c. Exposure to bacterial endotoxins.
      4. Have half-time in blood of 6 hours. Migrate to spleen, liver, lung, and, to a lesser extent, gastrointestinal (GI) tract and oropharynx.
      5. Accumulation of neutrophils at sites of inflammation stimulated by:
         a. Lactoferrin.
         b. Neutrophil secretions.

    c. Chemotactic peptides.
6. Reach perivascular space by emigration. Once in tissue, migrate via chemotaxis.
7. Concentrate in large numbers at sites of infection. In rats, 10% total number of circulating neutrophils will accumulate per day in sites of infection.
8. Phagocytosis.
    a. Coating with opsonins enhances phagocytosis. Opsonins are:
      (1) Components of complement.
      (2) Gamma-globulin.
      (3) Other polypeptides.
    b. Can lead to death of leukocyte.

Radiopharmaceuticals

  I. Labeling technique—Indium-111 (^{111}In).
    A. Cell separation.
      1. ^{111}In tags all cell types indiscriminately; therefore, necessary to separate leukocytes from remainder of blood before labeling.
      2. For clinical studies, mixed cell preparations adequate. These contain variable number of lymphocytes, monocytes, eosinophils, red blood cells (RBCs), and platelets in addition to neutrophils. In experimental abscesses, no difference in concentrating ability is found between pure neutrophil preparations and mixed cell suspensions.
      3. Usual separation technique for obtaining mixed leukocyte population is gravity sedimentation. To hasten sedimentation, settling agents—hydroxyethyl starch—can be used.
      4. Leukocyte-rich supernatant contains as many as 70% of leukocytes in sample. Most of the platelets and one to two RBCs per leukocyte contaminate supernatant.
      5. Centrifugation done to:
        a. Reduce number of platelets in buffy coat.
        b. Reduce amount of plasma, step necessary for oxine labeling.
    B. Labeling.
      1. Oxine.
        a. Most commonly used labeling agent. Lipophilic ligand chelates bivalent and trivalent metal ions, such as ^{111}In.
        b. Plasma must first be removed by centrifugation since ^{111}In has higher affinity for plasma transferrin than for oxine.
        c. Leukocyte incubated with ^{111}In oxine. Oxine allows indium to enter cell. Bond then broken. ^{111}In binds intracellularly and oxine leaves the cell.

    d. Cells are then washed and recentrifuged to remove unbound oxine and ^{111}In oxine from preparation.
  2. Tropolone.
    a. Another chelating agent commonly used. May allow earlier imaging.
    b. Can label in plasma.
II. Quality control—^{111}In.
  A. Microscopic examination of leukocytes to look for damage.
  B. Check labeling efficiency. E = C/C + W × 100 where C indicates activity associated with cells; W, activity associated with wash; and E, labeling efficiency.
III. Radiation effects—^{111}In.
  A. Neutrophil receives 1,480 rad when blood labeled with 1 mCi of ^{111}In.
  B. Studies indicate leukocytes receiving up to 50,000 rad external radiation show normal phagocytic and metabolic function.
  C. Radiation-induced oncogenesis.
    1. Neutrophils, postmitotic cells, are relatively radioresistant. Oncogenesis not a problem.
  D. Lymphocytes.
    1. 20 to 30 million of hundred million leukocytes labeled in typical mixed cell preparation will be lymphocytes.
    2. Labeled lymphocytes receive much higher radiation dose than neutrophils—8,750 rad. This is an essentially killing dose. Therefore, oncogenesis from irradiated lymphocytes is not considered a significant problem.
IV. Hexamethyl propyleneamine oxime (HMPAO).
  A. Labeling.
    1. A small, neutral, lipophilic complex that readily crosses cell membranes. When incubated with leukocytes, HMPAO enters cell and changes into a secondary hydrophilic complex that is trapped in cell. Activity is bound to intracellular organelles, especially nucleus and mitochondria.
    2. Labeling can be done in plasma.
    3. Labeling efficiencies of 37% to 86%.
    4. An almost pure granulocyte label.
      a. Predilection for polys.
      b. Tag of other cell types is not as stable and washes out.
    5. Labeled cells have normal function.

Imaging Technique

  I. Patient is given 500 µCi ^{111}In leukocytes injected IV.
  II. Leukocytes imaged 24 hours after injection.

III. Large-field-of-view camera with medium energy collimator using 173, 247-keV photopeaks with 20% windows.

IV. First image over liver/spleen with information density (ID) 500 to 700 over liver for minimum 200-K counts. Anterior and posterior images over abdomen, pelvis, and chest then done for same time as liver image. Images of extremities require increased time to obtain adequate film density.

V. Whole body imaging—dual-headed camera.

    A. Medium energy collimator.

    B. Energy settings as above.

    C. Matrix—256 × 1024.

    D. Image 50 minutes.

VI. Energy settings of camera changed to ^{99m}Tc.

VII. When leukocyte completed, patient injected with 5 mCi ^{99m}Tc sulfur colloid.

VIII. General all-purpose (GAP) collimator used for imaging.

IX. Standard liver/spleen scan performed.

X. This compared with leukocyte scan.

XI. Early imaging (1 to 4 hours after injection of leukocytes) can be done if necessary to make a rapid diagnosis. Sensitivity not as high as at 24 hours.

XII. ^{99m}Tc HMPAO leukocyte technique.

    A. Camera settings similar to whole body imaging for ^{111}In but with Tc collimator.

    B. Image at 1 to 4 hours. Early imaging allows evaluation of abdomen before normal bowel activity appears. Delayed imaging performed as needed.

Normal Scan

I. Thirty minutes to 4 hours after injection.

    A. Pulmonary uptake seen.

        1. Cause unknown. May be due to damage during labeling, which is then repaired in lungs, or may be due to physiologic margination in lungs' vasculature.

II. Twenty-four hours.

    A. Liver, spleen, bone marrow activity. Spleen highest activity, liver less, bone marrow least.

    B. No renal or GI activity normally seen.

III. ^{99m}Tc HMPAO leukocytes.

    A. Biodistribution varies significantly from ^{111}In labeled cells.

        1. Initial distribution is similar to ^{111}In. Uptake occurs in lungs, liver, and spleen.

2. Bladder and kidney activity is seen as early as 1 hour; gallbladder seen in 4% at this time.
3. By 4 hours lung activity falls, but gallbladder activity increases (10%) and bowel activity is seen.
4. At 24 hours, colonic activity is seen in all patients.
5. Gallbladder and bowel activity is thought to be due to excretion of secondary complex, as is seen with HMPAO brain imaging.
6. The genitourinary activity is *not* due to free pertechnetate; thyroid activity is not seen.

Abnormal Scans

I. Areas of uptake outside normal organs.
II. The greater the intensity of uptake when compared with liver, the greater the chance that an inflammatory lesion indicates infection.
  A. Activity equal to or greater than that of liver indicates infectious process.
  B. Activity significantly less than liver, more likely noninfectious process.

Findings

I. Abdominal abscess.
  A. Background—35% mortality for untreated abdominal abscesses.
    1. Frequently follow GI/genitourinary (GU) surgery.
  B. Leukocyte scan.
    a. Sensitivity—average 90%.
    b. Specificity—95%.
  C. Focal area of increased uptake usually greater than or equal to liver in intensity.
  D. Abscesses in liver may have same activity as remainder of liver. Will be detected when colloid liver/spleen scan (shows cold defect) compared to leukocyte scan.
II. Lung uptake.
  A. Less specific for infection than uptake in other areas. One sixth of scans show lung uptake.
  B. Diffuse uptake, infection only 10% of time.
  C. Focal uptake, infection 50% of time.
  D. Causes of lung uptake other than infection include:
    1. Congestive heart failure (CHF).
    2. Adult respiratory distress syndrome (ARDS).
    3. Atelectasis.
    4. Pulmonary emboli (PE).
    5. Aspiration.
    6. Idiopathic.
III. Gastrointestinal tract activity.

A. Nineteen percent of patients with fever of unknown origin show uptake in GI tract.
B. Correlates with cause of fever in only one half of patients.
C. Most common causes of true positives are:
  1. Abscess communicating with bowel.
  2. Pseudomembranous colitis.
  3. Inflammatory bowel disease.
  4. Necrotic bowel.
D. Most common causes of false-positive findings are:
  1. Swallowed leukocytes.
    a. Long-term in-dwelling endotracheal, Dobhoff, and other tubes, which cause significant inflammation.
    b. Pneumonia and empyema.
    c. Sinusitis.
  2. Bleeding.
    a. Ulcers.
    b. Diverticula.
    c. Tumors.
IV. Other "normal" sites of uptake:
A. IV catheters.
B. Colostomies.
C. Uninfected postsurgical wounds (10 days old or less).
D. Hematomas.
E. Accessory spleen.

Other Considerations

I. Imaging time.
A. Sensitivity for abscesses when imaging 1 to 4 hours after injection—30% to 50% when compared with 24-hour imaging. Better results early reported by some investigators using different chelating agent—tropolone—rather than oxine.
B. ^{99m}Tc HMPAO leukocytes.
  1. Sensitivity is near maximum at 30 to 60 minutes.
II. Low white blood cell counts.
A. Neutropenic patients frequently develop abscesses, yet often without localizing signs.
B. Patients have insufficient number of leukocytes for labeling.
C. Donor cells, ABO matched, can be used.
D. Sensitivity of donor cells equal to autologous cells.
E. Occasional problems with granulocyte-agglutinating antibodies to transfused leukocytes.
III. Chronicity of infection.
A. Might expect decreased infiltration of neutrophils in sites of chronic infection (>2 weeks.).

B. However, studies show leukocytes have similar sensitivity for acute and chronic infections. Possible explanations include:
1. Significant neutrophil infiltration occurs in chronic *bacterial* infections.
2. Some labeled lymphocytes may migrate to sites before they die.
C. ^{99m}Tc HMPAO leukocytes.
1. May not be as sensitive in chronic infection. Exchange of leukocytes is slowed in these sites and delayed imaging of up to 24 hours may be required.
IV. Effect of antibiotics.
A. Could decrease leukocyte chemotaxis by:
1. Killing bacteria, thereby preventing elaboration of chemotaxins.
2. Direct negative effect on leukocyte itself.
B. No significant effect found on sensitivity of leukocyte scan has been shown, however.
V. Spinal infections.
A. Evidence that labeled leukocytes are not as sensitive for spinal infections. Reason is not known.
VI. Comparison with gallium 67 (^{67}Ga).
A. Animals.
1. In dogs, abscess concentration of ^{111}In leukocytes is approximately 50 times greater than ^{67}Ga.
B. Humans.
1. Sensitivities of tests similar—90% gallium, 96% indium.
2. However, specificity of indium much higher—98%—than gallium—64%.
VII. Use of radiographic procedures to diagnose abscesses.
A. Choice of computed tomography (CT), ultrasound, ^{111}In leukocytes for abscess detection. Recommended order of use:
1. Patients with no localizing signs and low clinical suspicion of abscess—^{111}In leukocyte scan. 20% of sites of infection outside abdomen in these patients. Obviously would be missed by ultrasound and CT.
2. No localizing signs and high clinical suspicion of abscess.
a. Begin with ^{111}In leukocyte scan. *If negative,* do second modality.
3. Patients with localizing signs or extremely ill patients.
a. CT (ultrasound second choice) gives immediate answer. If these negative, follow with ^{111}In leukocyte scan.
VIII. The choice of ^{99m}Tc HMPAO versus ^{111}In leukocytes.
A. ^{99m}Tc HMPAO leukocytes are preferred in:

   1. Acute sepsis in which a rapid answer is needed.
   2. Musculoskeletal infection (especially in extremities), in which high photon flux is helpful.
B. ^{111}In leukocytes.
   1. Fever of unknown origin.
   2. Chronic infection.
   3. Gastrointestinal and genitourinary inflammation.

Radiolabeled Antibodies for Infection Imaging

I. Background.
   A. Two approaches—monoclonal and polyclonal antibodies.
   B. Monoclonal antibodies.
      1. Can be whole antibodies or Fab' fragments.
      2. Aimed against an antigen on leukocyte cell surface.
      3. Do not require in vitro manipulation to label leukocytes.
      4. Because they are a murine antibody, they cause recipient to develop human antimouse antibodies in 10% to 40%. Note: Whole antibodies are more likely to produce HAMAs; Fab' fragments appear less likely to do so.
      5. Sensitivities of 95% have been reported.
      6. Specificity is somewhat lower because both infectious and non-infectious causes of inflammation will show uptake.
         See discussion at end of chapter for more background information about monoclonal antibodies.
   C. Polyclonal antibodies.
      1. Mechanism of uptake in sites of inflammation is not well understood. Proposed mechanisms of uptake include:
         a. Increased vascular permeability.
         b. Binding to Fc receptors on granulocytes.
         c. Binding to bacteria.
         d. Physicochemical reaction.
         e. Carrier protein and radiolabel chemistry.
      2. Do not produce HAMAs.
      3. Effective with both bacterial and nonbacterial agents.
      4. Sensitivities of 97% to 100% have been reported.
      5. Specificity is somewhat lower because these are nonspecific markers of inflammation rather than being specific markers of infection.

RADIOLABELED PLATELETS
Anatomy and Physiology

   I. Platelets formed in bone marrow by megakaryocytes.
  II. Small disk-shaped cells; do not have nucleus.

Table 8-1   Radiolabels

Radioisotope	Half-Life (Days)	Gamma Energy (KeV)
Indium 111	2.7	172, 247
Chromium 51	27.0	320

III. Have ability to change shape on contact with foreign materials or subendothelial surfaces stimulating release of substances involved in hemostasis.
IV. Hemostasis.
   A. Platelet adhesion to periphery of wound.
   B. Localized vasoconstriction.
   C. Platelet plug formation.
   D. Reinforcement of plug with fibrin.
   E. Removal of clot by fibrinolytic system.
V. Prostaglandins.
   A. When platelets are activated, convert arachidonic acid to endoperoxidases and thromboxane-A_2. Thromboxane A_2 is one of most potent vasoconstrictors known. Also promotes platelet aggregation. Prostacyclin, produced in vessel wall, inhibits thromboxane effect. Aspirin and other drugs that decrease platelet aggregation do so by inhibiting cyclooxygenases. This blocks conversion arachidonic acid to peroxidase, reducing thromboxane A_2 levels.

Technique

I. Labeling.
   A. Two types of platelet labels:
      1. Cohort (pulse) labels—taken up by megakaryocytes and incorporated into components of forming platelets. With these labels, only freshly released platelets of uniform age are tagged. Not clinically used at present.
      2. Random labels—tag all ages of platelets in peripheral blood. Chromium 51 chromate and indium 111 oxine are examples (Table 8-1).
   B. Collection of blood.
      1. Anticoagulant used in blood-collecting syringe critical. ACD has much less deleterious effect on platelets' function than do other anticoagulants.
   C. Centrifugation.
      1. Two steps.
         a. First centrifugation at 1,750 to 2,700 g/minute produces platelet-rich plasma (PRP).

(1) Higher forces, too many platelets lost. Lower forces, excessive RBC contamination.

(2) Duration of centrifugation also important—as increase time, younger platelets that are more adhesive tend to sediment out.

b. Centrifugation (10,000 to 20,000 g/minute) of PRP forms platelet pellet, removing plasma.

B. Indium 111 oxine.

1. Because of physical characteristics, ^{111}In superior to ^{51}Cr as platelet label (Table 8-1).

2. Labeling in plasma, although reducing labeling efficiencies, may improve function.

C. Other chelates.

1. Other agents that may have less toxic effect on platelets include:

a. Tropolone

b. 2-Mercaptopyridine-N-oxide.

II. Radiation effects.

A. 12,900 rad to individual platelet incubated with 1 mCi of ^{111}In. High value due to relatively small size and long biologic life span.

B. Since lack nucleus, are highly radioresistant. Normal survival times and function reported at radiation doses of 50,000 to 70,000 rad.

Clinical Uses

I. Platelet survival studies.

A. One of most common uses of radiolabeled platelets is to measure platelet life span.

B. Survival curve normally linear. Disappearance of platelets from circulation is related to age-dependent destruction by reticuloendothelial (RES) system.

C. Life span normally equals 9 days.

D. Curves in normals may deviate from ideal in 2 ways.

1. Plateau at 48 hours.

a. Cause may be related to:

(1) Reversible liver sequestration of labeled platelets.

(2) Gradual fall in platelet-transit times through spleen with net shift of platelets out of splenic pool.

(3) Failure of older platelets to be labeled.

b. Prolonged tail may be formed 7 to 8 days. More common with chromium than with indium. May be related to preferential tagging of younger platelets when low chromium concentrations used.

E. Pathologic processes (nonlinear curve shapes).

1. Platelets survival diminished in number of conditions including:
     a. Idiopathic thrombocytopenic purpura (ITP).
     b. Prosthetic heart valves.
     c. Arterial grafts.
     d. Peripheral vascular disease.
     e. Atherosclerotic coronary heart disease.
     f. Eisenminger's syndrome.
     g. Primary pulmonary hypertension.
     h. Diabetes mellitus.
     i. Hepatic cirrhosis.
     j. Hyperlipidemia.
     k. Renal transplantation.
II. Deep venous thrombosis.
   A. In dogs—thrombus-to-blood ratios of 20 to 50 occur.
   B. Sensitivity—95%.
   C. Specificity—100% in some studies.
   D. Problems.
     1. In animals, heparin prevents visualization of thrombi. In humans, however, effect does not appear as significant.
     2. Degree of uptake dependent on thrombus age. Less localization in older thrombi.
     3. Delayed imaging 24 to 48 hours often necessary, especially in older thrombi.
III. Pulmonary embolism.
   A. Heparin appears to prevent embolus visualization.
   B. Amount of time thrombus present in lung important for sensitivity—not age of thrombus itself. With aging, in situ adherence of platelets to emboli diminishes.
   C. Large emboli that completely occlude artery may cause false-negative studies because emboli not exposed to labeled platelets in blood.
IV. Cerebrovascular disease.
   A. Evidence platelets involved in pathogenesis includes:
     1. Fibrin-platelet thrombi frequently found adhering to plaques at endarterectomy.
     2. Platelet emboli found in retinal vessels during amaurosis fugax.
   B. Results using radiolabeled platelets has been disappointing. Sensitivity for angiographically proven cerebrovascular disease average 50%. Reasons for low sensitivity include:
     1. Formation of platelet thrombi and plaques may be less impor-

tant than other factors in pathogenesis of cerebrovascular disease.

2. Platelet deposition may be occurring in foci too small to detect.
3. Antiplatelet and anticoagulation therapy may decrease uptake (although most studies indicated they have little effect).
4. Because a lesion is present anatomically does not mean it is physiologically active with platelets actively accumulating and being embolized.

BONE MARROW IMAGING
Anatomy and Physiology

I. Functional red marrow rivals liver in total size, weighing 1,500 g.
II. Distribution of active marrow.
   A. Adults—found primarily in:
      1. Axial skeleton including:
         a. Vertebral bodies.
         b. Pelvis.
         c. Sternum.
         d. Scapula.
         e. Skull—to a variable extent.
      2. Appendicular skeleton.
         a. Proximal one third of femora and humeri.
   B. Children.
      1. Extent dependent on age.
      2. Newborns—active marrow extends full length of extremities.
      3. As child grows, marrow gradually retracts until adult pattern reached at age 10.
III. When increase in RBC production needed:
   A. Erythroid marrow hypertrophies at expense of fat in marrow cavity. Because this occurs in skeleton normally containing active marrow, scintigraphy cannot detect these early changes.
   B. As production requirements increase, erythroid marrow moves peripherally in the long bones and even small bones of hands and feet. This abnormal distribution can be detected on marrow scan.

Radiopharmaceuticals

I. Radioiron and analogues.
   A. Bind to transferrin.
   B. Incorporated into active erythroid precursors in bone marrow.
   C. Eighty percent to 90% plasma iron turnover resulting from marrow erythropoiesis.
   D. Iron 52.

    1. Requires cyclotron for production.
    2. Half-life—8 hours.
    3. Best-quality images produced with positron camera.
  E. Iron 59.
    1. Photon energy—1.089, 1.298 meV.
    2. Specially built equipment with heavy collimation necessary.
    3. Half-life—45 days. Allows only small doses to be administered, which contributes to poor-quality images.
  F. Few institutions perform radioiron imaging for above reasons.
II. Reticuloendothelial system imaging.
  A. General characteristics.
    1. Colloids are removed from blood by phagocytic cells of RES that line bone marrow sinusoids.
    2. Normally, erythron and RES bound together; thus, RES scans show identical marrow distributions with radioiron.
    3. In most diseases both marrow components affected similarly.
    4. Occasionally, hematopoietic marrow may be absent at sites containing RES. Reverse, hematopoietic activity without associated RES, rare.
  B. Technetium 99m sulfur colloid.
    1. Ninety-two percent of IV dose removed by phagocytes of RES system in liver and spleen.
    2. Remaining 8% localizes in bone marrow.
    3. With usual dose of sulfur colloid used for liver spleen scanning and relatively short imaging times, activity in bone marrow not normally seen. Higher doses allow bone marrow to be visualized.
    4. Disparate imaging between sulfur colloid and radioiron.
      a. Disparate imaging is seen when increased marrow activity with peripheral expansion of RES, not blood-forming, erythropoietic marrow, occurs. Radioiron scan will *correctly* show diminished marrow uptake reflecting lack of erythropoietic marrow. Sulfur colloid will be normal or increased. Such disparity reported in:
        (1) Pure RBC aplasia.
        (2) DeGuglielmo's syndrome.
        (3) Hematologic malignancies.
        (4) Aplastic anemia.
        (5) Advanced myeloid metaplasia with myelofibrosis.
  C. Indium 111 chloride.
    1. Imaging characteristics.
      a. Decay—electron capture.
      b. Photon energy—173, 247 keV.

     c. Half-life—2.8 days.

  2. Physiology.

     a. Indium binds to transferrin similar to iron.

     b. Indium does not behave identically to iron, however.

     c. In rat, iron transported across placenta, whereas indium is not.

     d. Indium disappears more slowly from plasma than iron.

     e. Only 4% injected indium associated with circulating erythrocytes, compared with 80% injected radioiron.

     f. External radiation temporarily dissociates RES and erythroid function.

       (1) Diminished iron 59 uptake.

       (2) Sulfur colloid shows no change.

       (3) ^{111}In found to act similar to colloid (i.e., radiation does not significantly reduce uptake).

  3. Clinical use.

     a. Good correlation between ^{111}In scans and clinical status found in:

       (1) Aplastic anemia.

       (2) Myelofibrosis.

       (3) Variety of other hematologic disorders.

     b. Disparity with ^{111}In found in:

       (1) Some hypoplastic marrow diseases (e.g., RBC aplasia).

Technique

I. ^{99m}Tc sulfur colloid.

  A. Patient is injected with 12 to 15 mCi ^{99m}Tc sulfur colloid IV.

    1. Higher doses *not* given to saturate RES system to allow larger percentage of dose to be deposited in bone marrow. Within physiologically acceptable doses, cannot saturate RES system of liver and spleen.

    2. Higher dose is used so that 8% injected dose is enough activity to allow marrow to be visualized scintigraphically, using acceptable imaging times.

  B. Imaging performed with large-field-of-view camera using low-energy all-purpose (LEAP) collimator.

    1. Image 30 minutes to 1 hour after injection.

    2. Obtain 50-K to 200-K counts per image or 800 counts/sq cm.

    3. Entire body imaged both anteriorly and posteriorly.

II. Indium 111 chloride.

  A. Inject 1 to 2 mCi IV.

    1. In patients with saturated iron-binding capacities, injected ^{111}In may not bind to transferrin. Forms colloid that is subsequently

       phagocytized by RES system. Must preincubate with transferrin.

  B. Twenty-four to 48 hours later, begin imaging.

  C. Large-field-of-view camera with medium energy collimator. Photopeaks set 173, 247 keV with 20% windows.

  D. Use similar counting statistics to technetium.

  E. Whole body imaged.

Normal Scan

  I. ^{99m}Tc sulfur colloid.

    A. Majority of uptake in the axial skeleton.

    B. Activity in appendicular skeleton should not extend beyond proximal one third.

    C. In children, extent varies with age—see above.

    D. Skull—variable degree of uptake.

    E. Sternum and ribs—often difficult to visualize although contain active marrow.

    F. Lower thoracic/upper lumbar region of spine not well seen because of intense uptake of liver and spleen.

  II. ^{111}In.

    A. Similar findings to RES except:

      1. Much less intense liver and spleen activity.

      2. Renal activity.

  III. Radioiron.

    A. Activity confined primarily to axial skeleton.

    B. Not normally accumulated in spleen.

Abnormal Scans

  I. Abnormalities seen on scan:

    A. Decreased central marrow.

    B. Peripheral extension.

    C. Focal defects.

    D. Increased liver and spleen size.

    E. Increased uptake outside normal regions extramedullary hematopoiesis.

  II. Clinical uses.

    A. Avascular necrosis (AVN).

      1. Background.

        a. Plain films normal for first 6 months in AVN.

        b. Bone scan normal 48 hours following subcapital fracture. Then decreased activity for a variable period, followed by increased activity in reparative phase. Thus bone scan difficult to interpret.

Table 8-2   Grading System for Colloid Hip Studies

Grade	Activity in Femoral Head	Interpretation
−	Less than adjacent background	Absent circulation
±	Equal to background	Minimum circulation
+	Progressively greater	Adequate circulation
++	than background	
+++	activity	
++++		

c. When blood supply to femoral head interrupted, marrow cells are first cells to die; therefore, marrow scan very sensitive early in course of the disease.

d. ^{99m}Tc sulfur colloid usual agent.

   (1) Ten mCi injected IV.

   (2) Patients imaged 1 to 2 hours later over hips.

   (3) Graded in activity from 1 to 4+ (Table 8-2). Important for patient to have hips internally rotated. Otherwise, false-negatives may occur if normal greater trochanter activity superimposes on cold head.

   (4) If hip has 1+ or greater activity, considered adequate flow to sustain head.

   (5) Zero, or especially minus activity, most significant.

   (6) Accuracy—95%.

e. Age-related findings:

   (1) Amount active marrow in hips diminishes with age.

   (2) Decline:

      (a) 11- to 19-year-olds—100% bilateral femoral head uptake.

      (b) 70 to 79—37% bilateral uptake.

   (3) Thus, unilateral AVN easier to diagnose than bilateral.

B. Extramedullary hematopoiesis.

  1. Background.

   a. Occurs in a number of diseases:

     (1) Chronic hemolytic anemias—thalassemia, sickle cell (SS) anemia, hereditary spherocytosis.

     (2) Myelophthisic anemias.

     (3) Myeloproliferative disorders—postpolycythemic myeloid metaplasia.

  2. Sites of occurrence.

   a. Liver and spleen—most common.

   b. Adrenal glands.

    c. Retroperitoneal fat.

    d. Lymph nodes.

    e. Renal pelvis.

    f. Breasts.

    g. Pleura.

    h. Falx cerebri.

    i. Lungs.

3. Clinical reasons for determining sites of extramedullary hematopoiesis.

    a. Determine if mass lesions seen on x-ray are due to extramedullary hematopoiesis rather than tumor.

       (1) Especially useful in intrathoracic masses.

       (2) Uptake by marrow agent indicates mass site of extramedullary hematopoiesis.

4. Since full bone marrow complement (including erythroid RES and megakerocytic cells) present in sites of extramedullary hematopoiesis, both RES and erythropoietic agents useful.

5. With ^{111}In, varying degrees liver-spleen activity seen in myelofibrosis that does not correlate well with presence erythropoietic elements. Uptake is due to phagocytosis by RES system of indium-colloid, which frequently forms.

C. Determine presence and contribution of splenic erythrocytosis in patients being considered for splenectomy in myeloproliferative disorders such as myeloid metaplasia.

1. Splenectomy—splenic ablation required because of pain caused by massive splenomegaly or hypersplenism.

2. Relative distribution of marrow, both intramedullary and splenic, determined with scan. Estimate if enough residual active marrow present to allow splenic site of extramedullary hematopoiesis to be removed.

D. Evaluate disparity between patient's marrow histology and peripheral blood smear.

1. Seen most commonly in patients with hypoplastic anemias whose marrow suggests more severe disease than would be expected from complete blood cell counts. Marrow scan helpful in:

    a. Determining if marrow sampling errors occurred.

    b. Determining best site from which to obtain second marrow sample.

2. Type of marrow agent to use is controversial. Because of disparity problems, erythropoietic agents best. ^{111}In good second choice.

E. Diagnosing bone marrow infarcts and hemolytic anemias.

1. Background.

      a. Marrow infarcts common in patients with SS anemia and variants (SC- and S-thalassemia).

      b. More than one half of patients with SS anemia have bone marrow infarcts at some time during course of disease.

      c. Infarctions caused by intravascular and intrasinusoidal sickling that causes hemopoietic marrow to become ischemic. Marrow necrosis causes deep bone pain that is characteristic of the disease.

      d. Over period of months to several years marrow repopulates in some sites while progressive to permanent fibrosis in others.

      e. Joint pain and swelling common. May be due to:

         (1) Microvascular occlusion in synovium.

         (2) Periarticular bone marrow infarction.

      f. Plain films usually normal in acute marrow infarctions.

      g. Sensitivity—very sensitive means for determining bone or joint symptoms due to marrow infarction.

  2. Technetium sulfur colloid.

      a. Because RES expands with hematopoietic marrow and hemolytic anemias, physical characteristics of technetium allow high-resolution imaging that improve sensitivity for small infarctions.

  3. Findings.

      a. Cold areas surrounded by increased uptake in surrounding active marrow.

      b. Most evident where marrow expansion present.

      c. Half of asymptomatic patients will show defects on marrow scan caused by previous infarction and fibrosis. Can cause false-positive findings.

  4. Bone scan not useful in differentiating infarction from osteomyelitis.

      a. Each disease can cause cold defects.

      b. Bone infarcts can become hot within days.

      c. Indium leukocytes or gallium best approach.

F. Detecting metastases.

  1. Background.

      a. Bone and bone marrow share common blood supply.

      b. Approximately 40% total blood flow to bone is to marrow.

      c. Tumors with propensity to metastasize to bone often have marrow involvement as well.

      d. Sensitivity.

         (1) Marrow imaging only increases yield over bone scanning alone by 5%.

        (2) Normal bone marrow scan in face of positive bone scan occurs 22% of the time.

        (3) Marrow scan has difficulty detecting metastases in skull, ribs, and extremities, where variable amount of bone marrow present normally.

        (4) Has been shown to be useful in neuroblastoma and multiple myeloma, however.

    e. Specificity.

        (1) False-positive findings more common with bone marrow scans than conventional bone scans. May be related to depression of marrow function via chemotherapy and radiation therapy.

        (2) Marrow defects may persist even with the eradication of disease, because of necrosis or fibrosis.

    f. Agent.

        (1) ^{99m}Tc sulfur colloid.

           (a) High-resolution images.

           (b) As added bonus, allows liver and spleen to be evaluated for metastases.

G. Diagnosis and staging of diffuse hematologic disorders.

  1. Polycythemia vera.

    a. Early—normal or minimal peripheral expansion.

    b. Ten percent to 20% of polycythemia vera patients, progress to myelofibrosis with myeloid metaplasia. Marrow scan shows generalized hypoplasia with some degree of peripheral expansion.

  2. Myelofibrosis.

    a. Decreased central activity resulting from replacement of axial marrow.

    b. In one half of patients with hyperplasia, causes peripheral expansion.

  3. Aplastic anemia.

    a. Little or no uptake in any region of skeleton.

    b. With recovery, scan reverts to normal central uptake with varying degrees of peripheral expansion.

  4. Hemolytic anemias.

    a. Peripheral expansion when anemia present for several weeks/months.

  5. Leukemia.

    a. Early or mild involvement—normal.

    b. With more significant involvement—decreased central marrow activity with packing of marrow space with blast cells.

    c. If associated with anemia or infection, variable degree of peripheral expansion.

6. Hodgkin's disease/lymphoma.
   a. Wide variation of marrow patterns.
   b. Most common finding—central marrow hyperplasia.
   c. Focal defects—20%.

MONOCLONAL ANTIBODIES FOR DETECTING TUMOR

I. Background.
   A. Antibodies are usually murine monoclonal antibodies produced in hybridomas.
   B. Biodistribution of murine antibodies in humans is, in general, dose dependent. With increasing dose:
      1. Prolonged serum $T_{1/2}$.
      2. Relatively increased tumor uptake.
      3. Relatively decreased visceral uptake.
      4. Mechanism of dose effect is likely due to increased saturation of antibody binding in liver and other nonspecific sites.
   C. Radiotracer metabolism.
      1. Indium label is better retained in tumor and tissues while iodine is more rapidly dehalogenated and excreted in urine. Indium and other tags, therefore, usually yield better target-to-background ratios than iodine.
   D. The presence of target or cross-reacting antigen may significantly shorten specific antibody $T_{1/2}$.
   E. Distribution of monoclonal antibodies is also dependent on route of administration. Lymphatic or intracavitary routes vary from IV distribution.

II. Clinical utility.
   A. Large number of monoclonal antibodies have been developed for prostate, ovarian, colorectal, breast, melanomas, etc. Most are being evaluated for clinical utility.
   B. In-111 labeled Mab B72.3—example of first FDA approved monoclonal antibody.
      1. Background.
         a. Localizes to tumor associated antigen (TAG-72), a high molecular weight glycoprotein expressed differentially by adenocarcinomas.
         b. In vitro studies indicate antibody is immunoreactive with 83% of adenocarcinomas, 97% of ovarian carcinomas, and the majority of breast, non–small-cell lung, pancreatic, gastric, and esophageal cancers.
      2. Technique.
         a. 1 mg antibody infused IV over 5 minutes, tagged to 5 mCi of In-111.
         b. Routine imaging at 48 and 72 hours.

c. Imaging performed with large-field-of-view camera with medium energy collimator and energy windows set at 173 and 247 keV.

d. SPECT performed as needed.

3. Normal biodistribution.

   a. Localizes in liver, spleen, bone marrow and blood pool. May also see activity in bowel, kidneys, bladder, male genitalia, and female nipples.

4. Findings.

   a. Increased uptake in tumor.

5. Sensitivity and specificity.

   a. Colorectal cancer.

      (1) Sensitivity of CT and Mab—69% vs 68%.

      (2) Mab more sensitive in pelvis—74% vs 57%.

      (3) CT more sensitive in liver—84% vs 41%.

      (4) Combined CT and Mab—88%.

      (5) Specificities of CT and Mab were equal—77%.

   b. Ovarian cancer.

      (1) Sensitivity Mab vs CT—59% vs 29%.

      (2) Note: Some benign ovarian tumors express TAG-72 antigen; therefore, scan cannot distinguish benign from malignant disease.

SCHILLING'S TEST
Physiology

I. B_{12} is not synthesized by plants or animals. It is produced by microorganisms found in soil and intestines and rumens of animals. Dietary B_{12} comes from meat and dairy products.

II. B_{12} primarily stored in liver.

III. Total body stores are high and daily excretion low. Takes 3 to 5 years to develop B_{12} deficiency if dietary intake halted or malabsorption occurs. Thus, B_{12} deficiency caused by diet is rare (unlike folate), occurring in strict vegetarians.

IV. For absorption, B_{12} must complex with intrinsic factor (IF). IF is protein secreted by parietal cells of gastric fundus.

V. B_{12}-IF complex moves down bowel and absorbed in terminal ileum. Requires alkaline pH and calcium. Complex dissociates, B_{12} diffuses or is actively transported across mucosa.

VI. B_{12} enters portal vein. Binds to transcobalamin-II transport protein. Delivers B_{12} to liver.

VII. Over next 8 to 12 hours, portion B_{12} reenters circulation binding to larger transport protein, transcobalamin I.

VIII. When storage capacity of transcobalamin I exceeded, B_{12} excreted

Schilling's test.
IX. B$_{12}$ deficiency caused by two primary mechanisms:
   A. Decreased intrinsic factor.
      1. Pernicious anemia—autoimmune.
      2. Gastrectomy.
   B. Intestinal malabsorption.
      1. Terminal ileum.
         a. Short bowel syndrome.
         b. Sprue.
         c. Regional enteritis.
         d. Lymphoma.
   C. Pancreatic.
      1. Chronic pancreatitis.
      2. Cystic fibrosis.
   D. Medications.
   E. Tape worm infestation.

Background

I. Clinical manifestations.
   A. Megaloblastic anemia—may be absent early in disease.
      1. Because of close metabolic relationship of vitamin B$_{12}$ and folate, folate administration can correct anemia. Unfortunately, neurologic change is unaffected and can progress. For this reason, important to differentiate folate from B$_{12}$ deficiency rather than simply using response to therapy.
   B. Thrombocytopenia.
   C. Leukopenia.
   D. Subacute combined degeneration of spinal cord.
      1. Note: Although hematologic change is reversible, neurologic may not be.

Radiopharmaceuticals

 I. Vitamin B$_{12}$ (cyanocobalamin) has cobalt as central metal atom. Radioactive isotopes of cobalt are substituted for cold atom, producing tagged form.
II. Radionuclides available:
   A. Cobalt 57.
      1. Decay—electron capture.
      2. Physical half-life—270 days.
      3. Photon energies—122 keV.
   B. Cobalt 58.
      1. Decay—electron capture, beta+, gamma.
      2. Physical half-life—71 days.

2. Physical half-life—71 days.
3. Photon energies—810 keV.

Technique

I. Part 1 of Schilling's test.
   A. Prepare dose standards—2 ml.
   B. Patient has nothing by mouth past midnight.
   C. Administer 0.5 μCi of ^{57}Co labeled vitamin B_{12} in 0.5 μg vitamin B_{12} orally.
   D. Two hours later, administer 1,000 μg of cold vitamin B_{12} intramuscularly or subcutaneously.
      1. Administered to saturate transport proteins.
   E. Collect two consecutive 24-hour urine collections.
      1. ^{57}Co vitamin B_{12} absorbed through GI tract will not be bound by saturated transport proteins and will thus be excreted in urine.
   F. Measure volume for 24-hour collection.
   G. Pipette and count 2-ml aliquots of urine and dose standards.
   H. Calculate percent of administered dose excreted over each 24-hour period.
II. Part 2 of Schilling's test.
   A. Repeat examination with 0.5 μCi ^{57}Co-labeled vitamin B_{12} complexed to human intrinsic factor.

Normal Findings

I. Part 1.
   A. Greater than 10% administered dose excreted in urine in first 24 hours. Values of 6% to 10% indeterminate.

Abnormal Findings

I. Pernicious anemia.
   A. Part 1.
      1. Less than 6% excreted. Usually much lower, 1% to 3% range.
   B. Part 2.
      1. Decreased part 1 result corrected to normal. Excretion greater than 10%.
   C. Chronic vitamin B_{12} deficiency from pernicious anemia can produce atrophy of ileal mucosa. Causes decreased intestinal absorption of B_{12}. In these cases, only minor correction in part 2. To diagnose this, repeat part 2 several weeks or months after institution of B_{12} therapy to allow mucosa to recover.
   D. False-positive results may occur in patients with diminished renal function or obstruction. Percent excreted in second 24-hour sample should be added to first. If combined excretion in normal

range, test interpreted as normal. In patients with extremely poor renal function, 3-day collection should be performed.
  E. False-positive if portion of urine volume lost. Maximum excretion 8 to 12 hours after administration. Can check for loss by:
    1. Measuring urine specific gravity.
    2. Creatinine—normally greater than 1 g.
    3. Differences in volume between 24- and 48-hour collections.
II. Intestinal malabsorption.
  A. Part 1—less than 6% excretion.
  B. Part 2—less than 6% excretion.

RED BLOOD CELL SURVIVAL

Background

I. Test done to determine whether anemia caused by decreased survival of red blood cells (RBCs).

Technique

  I. Ten milliliters of blood collected in 1.5 ml of ACD.
  II. Blood centrifuged, plasma discarded.
  III. Remaining packed cells tagged with 0.5 µCi/kg chromium 51 chromate.
  IV. Cells washed and recentrifuged to remove any unbound ^{51}Cr.
  V. Volume restored by adding isotonic saline. Reinjected in patient.
  VI. Samples withdrawn beginning 24 hours later every other day for 21 days.
    A. Time zero sample cannot be obtained earlier than 24 hours because approximately 10% of label lost on the first day. May be due to:
      1. Normal accelerated elution.
      2. Damage during labeling.
  VII. Microhematocrit determined for each sample. Counting performed in a well counter.
  VIII. Blood counts plotted on semilog paper.
    A. Dividing whole blood cell counts by sample hematocrit improves accuracy. Corrects for daily fluctuations of hematocrit.

Normal Findings

I. Half-time—25 to 35 days.
  A. Normal RBCs have 120-day life span; 0.8% of RBCs lost through senescence per day.
  B. Measured ^{51}Cr RBC survival half-time not 60 days as predicted, because of additional 1% loss of elution of tag from RBCs.

Abnormal Findings

I. Less than 25- to 35-day survival.
  A. Patient must be in steady state. Recent hemorrhage or transfusion affects accuracy.
  B. If hematocrit varies significantly (patient not in steady state), closer approximation of RBC survival obtained by plotting whole blood cell counts without hematocrit correction.

SPLENIC SEQUESTRATION
Background

I. Performed to determine if destruction of RBCs, which causes shortened RBC survival, is caused by splenic destruction of RBCs.

Technique

  I. Usually performed in conjunction with RBC survival study.
 II. Imaging performed on same every-other-day schedule as RBC survival study.
III. Activity measured over precordium, anterior liver, and posterior spleen.

Normal Findings

  I. Spleen-to-liver ratio of 1:1.
 II. Ratio remains approximately 1:1 over course of study.

Abnormal Findings

  I. Increased spleen-to-liver ratio.
 II. Increasing spleen-to-liver ratio over course of study.
  A. Splenomegaly itself, without pathologic sequestration, can yield spleen-to-liver ratios of 2:1 to 4:1. For this reason, rising ratio best evidence of significant sequestration.

RED BLOOD CELL VOLUME
Background

 I. Most common reason for performing these studies is to differentiate stress polycythemia from polycythemia vera.
II. Polycythemia vera.
  A. Characterized by overproduction of RBCs, often increased white blood cells and platelets as well. Increased blood viscosity causes:
    1. Stroke.
    2. Myocardial infarction.
    3. Venous thrombosis.
    4. Hemorrhage.

Technique

I. Background—based on dilution technique. Given amount tracer allowed to equilibrate with the space being measured, then sample obtained. By comparing quantity of administered tracer with concentration of tracer in sample, volume obtained. This expressed mathematically as:

$$P_v \text{ (ml)} = \frac{D_v \text{ (/ml) } D_c \text{ (cpm/ml)}}{P_c \text{ (cpm/ml)}}$$

D_v = volume dose given; D_c = concentration dose given; P_c = concentration tracer in pool to be measured; P_v = volume pool to be measured.

II. Technique.
   A. Draw 10 ml of blood.
   B. Incubate with μCi chromium 51 chromate.
   C. Centrifuge labeled blood at 1,000 g for 10 minutes.
   D. Discard plasma.
   E. Wash with saline and recentrifuge to remove unbound ^{51}Cr.
   F. Resuspend in saline.
   G. Make counting standard.
   H. Have patient in recumbent position 30 minutes.
      1. Blood volume varies with body positions. Supine is "standard" position.
   I. Inject 5 ml of labeled cells. From opposite arm draw 5-ml samples at 10 and 40 minutes.
      1. Samples at 10 and 40 minutes usually equal. If equilibration of RBCs delayed, such as in splenomegaly or polycythemia, 40 minutes more accurate than 10 minutes.
   J. Take 2 ml from sample and count. Perform microhematocrit.
   K. Calculate red cell volume (RCV) by:

$$RCV = \frac{\text{cpm/ml standard} \times (\text{HCT} \times .98) \times 1,000 \times 5}{\text{cpm/ml blood sample}}$$

   1. Correction of 0.98 necessary, since, when obtaining microhematocrit, some plasma trapped in RBC fraction.
   L. Blood volumes usually expressed as ml/kg. Because adipose tissue has lower total blood volume and RBC mass is compared with lean body tissue, can correct for ideal body weight.

Normal Findings

I. Males—25 to 35 ml/kg.
II. Females—20 to 30 ml/kg.

Abnormal Findings

I. Polycythemia vera.
   A. Males—greater than 36 ml/kg.
   B. Females—greater than 32 ml/kg.
   C. If extravasation of some cells occurs with reinjection, will calculate falsely higher RBC mass. Check for extravasation by comparing counts in injection site to opposite arm with hand-held monitor.
II. Stress polycythemia.
   A. Normal or reduced RBC mass.

PLASMA VOLUME
Background

I. Usually performed in conjunction with RBC mass. Used for diagnosis of polycythemia vera. Occasionally done for fluid balance.

Technique

I. Background—technique for measuring plasma volume similar to that for RBC mass. ^{125}I-labeled human serum albumin used as dilutional marker of plasma space. Because ^{125}I has 32-keV photon, plasma volume determination usually performed before RBC mass study.
II. Technique.
   A. Prepare a standard.
   B. Have patient rest in recumbent position 30 minutes.
   C. Draw 5 ml of blood.
   D. Centrifuge and remove 2 ml plasma and perform background count.
   E. Inject 5 µCi of ^{125}I human serum albumin.
   F. At 10 minutes draw 4 ml of blood.
   G. Centrifuge; remove 2 ml plasma and count.
   H. Plasma volume $= \dfrac{\text{cpm standard} \times 1000}{\text{cpm plasma sample}}$

Normal Findings

I. Males—30 to 45 ml/kg.
II. Females—30 to 45 ml/kg.

Abnormal Findings

I. Polycythemia vera.
   A. Usually normal.
   B. May be mildly increased or decreased.
II. Stress polycythemia vera.
   A. Diminished plasma volume.

B. Elevated hematocrit because of diminished plasma volume in face of normal RBC mass.

III. Normally, 9% of human serum albumin diffuses into extravascular space within first 10 minutes. In patients with diseases that increase protein loss or increase vascular permeability, greater amount of HSA may be lost. This gives falsely elevated plasma volume. More accurate plasma determination can be obtained in these patients by drawing additional samples at 20, 30, 60 minutes, then plotting and extrapolating back to time zero.

IV. Extravasation of injected dose, as in RBC volume determination, gives false values.

PHOSPHORUS 32 THERAPY FOR POLYCYTHEMIA VERA
Background

I. Three main forms of therapy for polycythemia vera.
   A. Phlebotomy—often combined with other two forms of treatment.
   B. Chemotherapy.
   C. Phosphorus (^{32}P) therapy.

Radiopharmaceutical

I. Phosphorus 32.
   A. Supplied as sodium phosphate.
      1. Pure beta emitter with average beta energy of 0.69 meV. This gives maximum 8-mm range (mean-3) in tissues. Because no accompanying gamma or x-radiation, isolation of patients not necessary.
      2. Low-energy bremstrahlung radiation occurs. Can be used to assay dose of ^{32}P.
   B. Action.
      1. Taken up by metabolically active tissues—highest concentraion in bone marrow and trabecular bone.
      2. Phosphates involved in many metabolic pathways. ^{32}P shows cellular proliferation by:
         a. Incorporation of ^{32}P into DNA with subsequent damage from emitted beta particles.
         b. ^{32}P decays to ^{32}S altering nucleic acid structure.
      3. Absorbed dose to marrow—20-50 rad/mCi. Average value approximately 24 rad/mCi.
         a. 13 rad—marrow uptake.
         b. 10 rad—trabecular bone.
         c. 1 rad—cortical bone.
   C. Dose.

1. Initial dose 2.3 mCi/sq m body surface area to maximum 5 mCi IV.
2. If 12 weeks later response inadequate, a repeat dose is given. Dose increased by 25% over previous one. Maximum, 7 mCi.
3. Regimen repeated for 1 year.

Complications

I. Acute leukemia.
   A. Controversial subject.
   B. Approximately 10% to 20% incidence with ^{32}P therapy compared to 1% phlebotomy alone. Chemotherapy—increased incidence of acute leukemia as well.
   C. Even with increased risk of leukemia, median survival with ^{32}P therapy 11 to 16 years compared with 7 to 8 years with phlebotomy alone. Without any therapy, median survival with polycythemia vera is 1.5 years.
II. Myelofibrosis with myeloid metaplasia.
   A. Probably not related to therapy. Is natural outcome of polycythemia vera in 10% to 20% of patients.

SUGGESTED READINGS

Bogard WC, Dean RT, Deo Y, et al: Practical considerations in the production, purification and formulation of monoclonal antibodies for immunoscintigraphy and immunotherapy. *Semin Nucl Med* 1989; 19:202-220.

Clarke-Pearson DL, Coleman RE, Petry N, et al: Postoperative pelvic vein thrombosis and pulmonary embolism detected by indium 111-labeled platelet imaging: A case report. *Am J Obstet Gynecol* 1984; 149:796-798.

Cook PS, Datz FL, Disbro MA, et al: Pulmonary uptake in indium-111 leukocyte imaging: Clinical significance in patients with suspected occult infections. *Radiology* 1984; 150:557-561.

Datz FL, Bedont RA, Baker WJ, et al: No difference in sensitivity for occult infection between tropolone- and oxine-labeled indium-111 leukocytes. *J Nucl Med* 1985; 26:469-473.

Datz FL, Jacobs J, Baker W, et al: Decreased sensitivity of early imaging with In-111 oxine-labeled leukocytes in detection of occult infection: Concise communication. *J Nucl Med* 1984; 25:303-306.

Datz FL, Luers P, Baker WJ, et al: Improved detection of upper abdominal abscesses by combination of ^{99m}Tc sulfur colloid and ^{111}In leukocyte scanning. *AJR* 1985; 144:319-323.

Datz FL, Morton KA: Radionuclide detection of occult infection: Current strategies. *Cancer Investig* 1991; 9:691-698.

Datz FL, Taylor A: Clinical use of radionuclide bone marrow imaging. *Semin Nucl Med* 1985; 15:239-259.

Datz FL, Taylor AT: Cell labeling: Techniques and clinical utility. In Freeman

LM (ed): *Freeman and Johnson's clinical radionuclide imaging.* New York, Grune & Stratton, 1984, pp 1785-1913.

Datz FL, Thorne DA: Effect of antibiotic therapy on the sensitivity of indium-111-labeled leukocyte scans. *J Nucl Med* 1986; 27:1849-1853.

Datz FL, Thorne DA: Effect of chronicity of infection on the sensitivity of the In-111-labeled leukocyte scan. *AJR* 1986; 147:809-812.

Datz FL, Thorne DA: Gastrointestinal tract radionuclide activity on In-111 labeled leukocyte imaging: Clinical significance in patients with fever of unknown origin. *Radiology* 1986; 160:635-639.

Davis HH, Siegel BA, Sherman LA, et al: Scintigraphy with ^{111}In-labeled autologous platelets in venous thromboembolism. *Radiology* 1980; 136:203-207.

Fischman AJ, Rubin RH, Khaw BA, et al: Detection of acute inflammation with ^{111}In-labeled nonspecific polyclonal IgG. *Semin Nucl Med* 1988; 18:335-344.

Goldenberg DM: Future role of radiolabeled monoclonal antibodies in oncological diagnosis and therapy. *Semin Nucl Med* 1989; 19:332-339.

Goldenberg DM, Goldenberg H, Sharkey RM, et al: Imaging of colorectal carcinoma with radiolabeled antibodies. *Semin Nucl Med* 1989; 19:262-281.

International Committee on Standardization in Haematology: Recommended methods for measurement of red-cell and plasma volume. *J Nucl Med* 1980; 21:793-800.

Joseph A, Hoffken H, Bosslet K, et al: In vivo labeling of granulocytes with ^{99m}Tc anti-NCA monoclonal antibodies for imaging inflammation. *Eur J Nucl Med* 1988; 14:353-367.

Peters AM, Roddie ME, Danpure HJ, et al: [99m]Tc HMPAO-labeled leukocytes: Comparison with ^{111}In-tropolonate-labeled granulocytes. *Nucl Med Comm* 1988; 9:449-463.

Powers WJ, Siegel BA: Thrombus imaging with indium-111 platelets. *Semin Thromb Hemost* 1983; 9:115-131.

Price DC, McIntyre PA: Hematopoietic system. In Harbert J, Goncalves de Rocha AF (eds): *Textbook in nuclear medicine. II: Clinical applications,* ed 2. Philadelphia, Lea & Febiger, 1984, pp 535-605.

Wright RR, Tono M, Pollycove M: Blood volume. *Semin Nucl Med* 1975; 5:63-78.

Zuckier LS, Chervu LR: Schilling evaluation of pernicious anemia: Current status. *J Nucl Med* 1984; 25:1032-1039.

Index

A

Abdominal abscess, radiolabeled leukocytes to diagnose, 236, 238
Ablation of thyroid in treatment of thyroid cancer, 22
Abscess(es)
  abdominal, radiolabeled leukocytes to diagnose, 236, 238
  amebic, 138
  brain, abnormal conventional planar studies in, 40
  liver, 115-116
  perinephric, 138-139
  renal, 164
  splenic, 119
  testicular, 183
Acalculous cholecystitis, acute, 124
Accelerated transplant rejection, 171
Acetazolamide test for vascular disease, 49-50
Acquired immunodeficiency syndrome, 139-140
Adenocarcinoma of head and neck, gallium imaging to diagnose, 142
Adenoma
  hepatic, 114
  hyperfunction, solitary, of thyroid, 19
  toxic, of thyroid, 19
Adenosine, pharmacologic stress produced by, 195, 200-201
Adrenal cortex
  anatomy of, 29
  imaging of, 29-32
    iodomethyl-19-norcholesterol for, 30
    radiopharmaceutical for, 30
  physiology of, 29
Adriamycin; see Cardiotoxicity
Advanced cirrhosis of liver, 118
Aerosols for pulmonary imaging, 91, 92
Agenesis of kidney, unilateral, 170
AIDS; see Acquired immunodeficiency syndrome

Albumin
  human, microspheres of, for pulmonary imaging, 89-90, 92-93
  ^{131}I human serum, for cerebrospinal fluid imaging, 54
  macroaggregated, for pulmonary imaging, 89-90, 92-93
Aldosteronism, 31-32
Aldosteronoma, 31
Alpha$_1$-antitrypsin deficiency, 102
Alzheimer's disease, 53
Amebic abscesses, 138
  of liver, 115-116
Americium 241 for thyroid scanning, 7-8
Amyloidosis, cardiac, 219
Anaplastic carcinoma of thyroid, 21
Androgen excess, 32
Anemia
  aplastic, bone marrow imaging to diagnose, 250
  hemolytic, bone marrow imaging to diagnose, 248-249, 250
  pernicious, 254-255
Aneurysmal bone cysts, 72
Aneurysms, 42
  ventricular, gated blood pool imaging to diagnose, 226-227
Angiogram
  cerebral; see Cerebral angiogram
  for Meckel's diverticulum, 129
  radionuclide, 37
Angiography, pulmonary, 95
Angiomyolipoma, renal, 168
Angiotensin II, 159
Angiotensin-converting enzyme, 159
Antibodies
  monoclonal, for detecting tumor, 251-252
  radiolabeled, for infection imaging, 239
Aplastic anemia, bone marrow imaging to diagnose, 250
Appendix epididymis, 178
  torsion of, 180, 181
Appendix testis, 178
  torsion of, 180, 181

BRITISH COLUMBIA CANCER AGENCY
LIBRARY
600 WEST 10th AVE.
VANCOUVER, B.C. CANADA
V5Z 4E6

6625   PO# 126720 $ 36.95 US